Praise for **The New Abnormal**

"Dr. Kheriaty documents how jumped-up technocrats abused power they never should have been granted and terrified people into surrendering their freedoms. The results of this malfeasance are both infuriating and ongoing. Fortunately, Kheriaty provides indispensable guidance for stopping an emerging biomedical security state from doing even more damage in the future."

 —**MOLLIE HEMINGWAY,** editor in chief of The Federalist, Fox News contributor, and author of the bestseller *Rigged: How the Media, Big Tech, and the Democrats Seized Our Elections*

"Dr. Kheriaty exposes the role of the biomedical security state behind the global response to the covid-19 pandemic. He offers helpful philosophical, psychological, and medical insights into the rise to power of this sinister cartel."

 —**ROBERT F. KENNEDY JR.,** author of *The Real Anthony Fauci: Bill Gates, Big Pharma, and the Global War on Democracy and Public Health*

"In his brilliant new book, Aaron Kheriaty brings together the expertise of a seasoned medical scientist, the wisdom of a true philosopher, and the acuity of a keen political observer. *The New Abnormal: The Rise of the Biomedical Security State* is must-reading for anyone who wants to understand how we have gone so wrong, and what we need to do now to chart a more humane path forward."

 —**RYAN T. ANDERSON,** author of *Tearing Us Apart* and president of the Ethics and Public Policy Center

"A sober reckoning is now upon us after the covid years. Dr. Aaron Kheriaty recounts how biomedical tyranny is born, his depiction amplified tenfold by descriptions of history's similar offenses against humanity. Kheriaty reminds us that there truly is nothing new under the sun. Maybe, just maybe, this time we'll heed that truth, remember, and change course. Our posterity deserves no less."

 —**JUSTIN HART,** founder of Rational Ground and author of *Gone Viral: How Covid Drove the World Insane*

"This book is both a masterwork and clarion call. The pandemic is over, but the threat of the response is still with us, revealing what we did not want to face, which is a problem that is ultimately philosophical. Do we believe in freedom anymore? If not, we'll go the way that he warns, straight to the hell of a biofascist security state. If this is not to be our fate, every person must engage in the intellectual battle for the future of the free society. This great work is essential to our understanding."

—**JEFFREY A. TUCKER**, founder and president of the Brownstone Institute

"Dr. Aaron Kheriaty has written an eye-opening, indeed frightening, account of a dystopian "biomedical security state"—the looming end point stemming from what was exposed by the SARS2 pandemic mismanagement debacle. When amplified by America's poisonous media influencing a public who trusted the "credentialed class" of public health and academia, the government imposed irrational lockdowns, school closures, and a host of mandates and restrictions that failed to stop the virus while inflicting massive damage and death on our most vulnerable—the elderly, low-income families, and our children. As Dr. Kheriaty details with authority, the most basic tenets of biomedical ethics, established for decades after an ugly history of actions purportedly in the name of medical science, were abandoned and remain in tatters today. This moral and ethical bankruptcy can in part be traced to what he exposes—the unholy cabal among the NIH, academia, harmful international organizations, and the biopharma industry that controls science research funding and careers. It behooves all good people to rise up—meaning stand up, speak up, as we are expected to do in free societies—to restore and preserve our most basic freedoms, and prevent 'The New Abnormal' Dr. Kheriaty warns about, before it is too late."

—**SCOTT W. ATLAS, M.D.**, senior fellow at the Hoover Institution at Stanford University, former adviser to the president's White House Coronavirus Task Force, and bestselling author of *A Plague upon Our House: My Fight at the Trump White House to Stop COVID from Destroying America*

"Over the past two years, very few medical ethicists have stood up to decry public health's violations of the basic principles of medical ethics, including informed consent, 'first do no harm,' and justice, so that the interests of the poor and vulnerable are not ignored. The lockdown policy adopted, 'The New Abnormal,' as Dr. Kheriaty memorably describes it, violated these principles, though so few have spoken up. The initial lockdowns themselves, including closed schools, businesses, and houses of worship, differentially harmed the young and the working class, even as covid spread despite them. When the vaccine became available, rather than relying on reasoned persuasion to encourage their uptake, American public health resorted to force in the form of discriminatory mandates and movement passes. All of these policies of The New Abnormal failed to protect people from covid and caused devastating collateral harm. It did not have to be this way. If we heed the lessons of this book, we can make sure that the next time there is a pandemic no one will think to establish a biomedical security state as a way to keep us safe from a virus when traditional public health and medical ethics practices would do a much better job."

—**JAY BHATTACHARYA**, professor of health policy at Stanford University

"*The New Abnormal* is required reading for the post-covid age. No mere spectator to the West's response to covid, Dr. Aaron Kheriaty placed himself on the frontlines, determined to save lives. But as Western leaders announced and repeatedly extended states of emergency and related coercive measures, Kheriaty, then a psychiatry professor and director of the medical ethics program at University of California at Irvine, found himself increasingly at odds with official policy—and many of his colleagues and friends. Digging deep into his varied expertise, in *The New Abnormal* Kheriaty describes a society hobbled by fear and groupthink, one increasingly on a technocratic, dehumanized path with an inevitably authoritarian bent. He then offers a powerful, hopeful framework to forestall the possible dystopian future he sees, complete with practical guidance any reader will benefit from. Beautifully written and engrossing."

—**JAN JEKIELEK**, senior editor at the *Epoch Times* and host of *American Thought Leaders*

The New Abnormal

THE NEW ABNORMAL
THE RISE OF THE BIOMEDICAL SECURITY STATE

Aaron Kheriaty, M.D.

Regnery Publishing
WASHINGTON, D.C.

Regnery® is a registered trademark and its colophon is a trademark of Salem Communications Holding Corporation

Cataloging-in-Publication data on file with the Library of Congress

ISBN: 978-1-68451-385-7
eISBN: 978-1-68451-388-8

Published in the United States by
Regnery Publishing,
A Division of Salem Media Group
Washington, D.C.
www.Regnery.com

Manufactured in the United States of America

10 9 8 7 6 5 4 3 2

Books are available in quantity for promotional or premium use. For information on discounts and terms, please visit our website: www.Regnery.com.

For my wife, Jennifer, who long ago perceived the dangers brewing: you resisted "the new normal" and you gave me courage to oppose it.

CONTENTS

Nuremberg, 1947

The principal office of history I take to be this: to prevent virtuous actions from being forgotten, and that evil words and deeds should fear an infamous reputation with posterity.

—*Tacitus*, Annals, *117 AD*

This book is about our future. But I begin with a cautionary tale from the not-so-distant past.

In the 1930s, German medicine and German health care institutions were widely considered the most advanced in the world. However, subtle but consequential shifts had been underway in German medicine and society for several decades. The process began long before Hitler came to power, starting with the rise of the eugenics movement in the early twentieth century. While the word eugenics is typically associated with Germany, and more specifically, with the atrocities of the Nazi regime, the eugenics movement began in the United States and Britain and was only later exported to Germany.

The idea of controlling population health by controlling reproduction started with the Anglo-American social Darwinists of the late nineteenth century. The term eugenics—defined as "the self-direction of human evolution"—was coined by Sir Francis Galton, Charles Darwin's cousin, who also coined the phrase "nature versus nurture." Writing of the superiority of eugenics over the achingly slow evolutionary process of natural selection, Galton wrote, "What nature does blindly, slowly, and ruthlessly, man may do providently, quickly, and kindly."[1] Eugenics was an effort to assume control over our human future by controlling who could or could not reproduce.

Although we now understand eugenics to be a pseudoscience based upon overly simplistic notions of trait inheritance, at the time it was considered a kind of master-science that brought together various scientific disciplines into a unified whole. The logo from the Second International Eugenics Congress in 1921 depicted the science of eugenics as a tree that unites many different fields from sociology and genetics to statistics, economics, biology, and psychology. Malthusian concerns about overpopulation, and well-intentioned (though deeply misguided) efforts to address social problems created by the Industrial Revolution, helped drive the eugenics movement.

The legalized practice of state-controlled breeding started in the United States. Beginning in 1907 and continuing until the 1970s, most states passed laws permitting the involuntary sterilization of those deemed "unfit" to reproduce. This resulted in sixty-five thousand forced sterilizations in thirty-three states. One-third of these occurred in my home state of California, where the practice continued until 1964. Most of these involuntary operations were endorsed by psychiatric physicians working in the system of state hospitals (a system in which I served as ethics committee chair from 2017 to 2021). Doctors served as the gatekeepers of forced sterilization.

Among the victims, Native Americans, blacks, Hispanics, immigrants, the mentally ill, the physically ill, and the poor were overrepresented. Women were involuntarily sterilized three times as often as men, even though tubal ligation is medically riskier and more invasive for women than vasectomy for men. The last forced sterilization under U.S. laws occurred in 1983. The regime continued even longer in the penal system: after revelations that dozens of women were forcibly sterilized in the California prison system between 2005 and 2011, the state finally passed a law banning this practice. A *Washington Post* headline in 2018 reported, "California Lawmakers Seek Reparations for People Sterilized by the State," many of whom were still alive.[2] This dark chapter in American history continued much longer than most Americans realize.

The forced sterilization laws in various states were typically based on Harry Laughlin's 1914 model legislation, which encompassed the "feebleminded," "insane," "criminalistic," "epileptic," "inebriate," "diseased," "blind," "deaf," "deformed," and "dependent," as well as "orphans, ne'er-do-wells, the homeless, tramps and paupers."[3] If many of these categories seem rather elastic from a medical or diagnostic perspective, I can confirm that "feeblemindedness" and "ne'er-do-wells" were categories no more clearly defined then than they are now.

Other eugenics-era public health policies entrenched racial discrimination and race-based exclusion. A Jim Crow–era article in the *Atlanta Constitution* newspaper claimed that "'the careless or ignorant Negro . . . is likely to nullify the scrupulous sanitary safeguards with which the white man surrounds his home and his business establishment' until there is one, strictly enforced, sanitary law for 'high and humble, Peachtree and Peters Street.'" We see this same racist condescension on display in popular print from the same era. For example, "The Negro cannot be interested in, nor can they readily understand the situation. They cannot be reached through regular channels, yet unless they are reached, treated and cured, they will continue to infect the soil and perpetuate the disease among the whites."[4] Public health experts mandated the rules they deemed necessary for people allegedly incapable of acting in their own or society's best interests.

Support for eugenics was mainstream in the United States. It was broadly embraced by the early twentieth-century progressive movement.[5] Eugenics programs received funding from major foundations, including those of Rockefeller, Carnegie, Ford, and Kellogg. Intellectuals at Stanford, Yale, Harvard, and Princeton endorsed the movement's aims and participated enthusiastically. David Starr Jordan, the founder of Stanford University, served as the first chair of American Breeder's Association. You could be forgiven for assuming that this association had something to do with dogs or horses; on the contrary, it was focused on the project of breeding better human beings. Jordan also penned a racist eugenics screed called *The Blood of the Nation* in 1902. Other outspoken eugenics advocates included Teddy Roosevelt, Margaret Sanger, Jack London, Alexander Graham Bell, Woodrow Wilson, Franklin Roosevelt (who explored a eugenic project to resettle Jews during World War II[6]), and, perhaps surprisingly given her disabilities, Helen Keller.

In the 1920s an impoverished young woman from Virginia, Carrie Buck, was diagnosed with "congenital feeblemindedness" and slated for forced sterilization. She challenged the state of Virginia's law in federal court, and her case, *Buck v. Bell*, went to the Supreme Court in 1927. The court upheld the state's eugenic sterilization law, resulting in Carrie's forced tubal ligation. Her younger sister was likewise involuntarily sterilized at the tender age of thirteen, after being told she was getting a surgery to remove her appendix.

Writing for the court's majority in this now infamous decision—a decision that the court has never officially overturned—the influential American jurist Oliver Wendell Holmes Jr. said: "It is better for all the world, if instead of waiting to execute degenerate offspring for crime, or to let them starve for their imbecility, society can prevent those who are manifestly unfit from continuing their kind. The principle that sustains compulsory vaccination is broad enough to cover cutting the Fallopian tubes." Holmes then concluded his argument in the court's majority decision by declaring that "three generations of imbeciles are enough."[7]

* * *

In 1933 Germany passed its own "Law for the Prevention of Hereditarily Defective Offspring," modeled on similar laws in the United States. Under their law Germany forcibly sterilized 350,000 citizens between 1934 and 1939, a far more relentless and efficient system than the one developed in the United States. With this groundwork laid, Germany took the logic of eugenics a step further. In 1922 a German psychiatrist and a German lawyer, Alfred Hoche and Karl Bidding, published an influential book titled *On the Destruction of Life Unworthy of Life*, an argument for involuntary euthanasia of those deemed unfit.

A metaphor from this book and other influential works captured the imagination of the German medical establishment, undermining the traditional Hippocratic ethic that had governed medicine since antiquity. Instead of serving the health of the individual patient presenting for treatment, German physicians were encouraged to be responsible for the health of the entire "social organism"—the *volk*, the people as a whole. This was a fateful—and fatal—shift in the ethics of medicine. The physician's loyalty was no longer primarily to the patient made vulnerable by illness or disability.

Instead of seeing the sick as individuals in need of compassionate medical care, German doctors became willing agents of a sociopolitical program driven by a cold utilitarian ethos. If the social organism was construed as healthy or sick, some individuals (for example, those with cognitive or physical disabilities) were characterized as "cancers" on the *volk*. And what do doctors do with cancers? They remove and eliminate them to preserve the health of the whole organism.

The idea of extending eugenics from forced sterilization to involuntary euthanasia was not, we should note, of wholly German extraction. Recall the American Breeder's Association mentioned above. In 1911 the Carnegie Foundation funded a study with the title *Preliminary Report of the Committee of the Eugenics Section of the American Breeder's Association to Study and Report on the Best Practical Means for Cutting off the Defective Germ-Plasm in the Human Population*. Germ plasm was the medical term of the day for the unknown biological mechanism of inheritance, prior to the discovery of DNA. Recommendation number 8 of this study, commissioned by a mainstream American foundation, was euthanasia.[8] Hitler himself remarked, "I have studied with interest the laws of several American states concerning prevention of reproduction by people whose progeny would . . . be of no value, or injurious to the racial stock."[9]

Soon after Hitler's rise to power in 1933, the Nazis promulgated the eugenics law mentioned above—modeled on the U.S. sterilization laws—"for the protection of the German people from hereditary diseases."[10] We should reflect carefully on this fact: the first case of legislation by which a nation-state programmatically assumed for itself the care of its citizens' health was that of Nazi eugenics. The first people gassed by the Nazis were not Jews in concentration camps (that came later) but disabled patients in psychiatric hospitals, killed without their consent under the Third Reich's T4 Euthanasia Program beginning in 1939.

Gas chambers, those hyperefficient technocratic mechanisms of mass killing, were not initially established by the Nazi government; they were initiatives of the German medical community. Like the involuntary sterilizations in the United States, each of the T4 euthanasia death warrants was signed by a German physician. Even after the lethal regime turned its attention on Jews and other ethnic minorities, the government continued to deploy quasi–public health justifications for the killing machine: the Jews were routinely demonized by the Nazis as "spreaders of disease."

This was the logical consequence of their fatal starting point. If physicians serve not the needs of sick and vulnerable patients, but are agents of a social program, the German example shows us what happens when that social program is misdirected by a corrupt regime. Conditioned by eugenic ideology, which had been prevalent for decades prior to Hitler, an alarming number of German physicians readily embraced Nazi doctrines. Although party membership was not a requirement of the medical profession, 45 percent of physicians voluntarily joined Nazi party; by comparison, only 10 percent of teachers joined.[11]

The actions of the Nazi doctors, particularly those who ran gruesome experiments on prisoners in concentration camps, were revealed at the postwar Nuremberg trials. The world rightly condemned the atrocities committed by German physicians and scientists. However uncomfortable, it is instructive to examine the defendants' arguments at the trials. Nazi doctors, who performed horrifying unconsented experiments on death camp prisoners, argued that nothing they had done was illegal under German law. This claim, it is sad to say, was true. To deal with this legal difficulty, the jurists at Nuremberg had to invoke the novel concept of "crimes against humanity"—a natural law argument that there are "some things you can't not know," and there are some "acts that can never be justified." That a physician or scientist was "just following orders" was not an adequate defense.

The defendants at Nuremberg also argued that prisoners in death camps were slated for extermination anyways, and many of them wanted to be selected for experimentation on the medical wards because the food-and-shelter conditions there were generally better than in the barracks. These claims were also true, though they likewise did not exonerate the defendants. Most notably, the defendants argued that the experiments were justified in the name of scientific progress and the greater good.

Many people today mistakenly assume that all Nazi medical experiments were simply quackery—an excuse for sociopaths like the infamous Josef Mengele to torment prisoners with impunity. While some of their experiments indeed had no plausible scientific value, more troublingly, useful experiments were conducted by most of the Nazi doctors. While it is uncomfortable to admit, real medical knowledge was gained that is still used today. Nazi doctors were particularly interested in applications to military medicine, trying to answer questions like, How long can a soldier shot down in the ocean survive before needing rescue? or, What happened physiologically to pilots at high altitudes?

Answers to these questions came by gruesome methods, including hypothermia experiments in which prisoners were placed in vats of ice water until they froze to death, or altitude experiments in which prisoners were placed in negative pressure chambers until their internal organs fatally exploded. Consult any embryology textbook today, and you'll find that it takes a fertilized human ovum three to four days to traverse the fallopian tube and implant in the uterus. You might wonder: How did we discover this? The answer is that Nazi doctors vivisected impregnated women.

At the 1946 Nuremberg trials, twenty-three physicians were indicted for crimes against humanity, sixteen were convicted, and seven of these received a death sentence and were executed in 1948. To prevent similar human rights disasters in the future, the central principle of research ethics and medical ethics—namely, the *free and informed consent of the research subject or the patient*—was clearly articulated in the Nuremberg Code in 1947. The first of the Code's ten principles begins:

> The voluntary consent of the human subject is absolutely essential. This means that the person involved should have legal capacity to give consent; should be so situated as to be able to exercise free power of choice, without the intervention of any element of force, fraud, deceit, duress, over-reaching, or other ulterior form of constraint or coercion; and should have sufficient knowledge and comprehension of the elements of the subject matter involved as to enable him to make an understanding and enlightened decision.[12]

While the Nuremberg Code did not enjoy the binding force of international law, its principles did inform the laws of most nations, including the United States. The principle of free and informed consent was further developed in the influential World Medical Association Declaration of Helsinki in 1964. This document specified additional safeguards for research on children who do not yet have decisional capacity to consent. It also drew attention to special populations—prisoners, disabled individuals, impoverished populations, et cetera—who require additional protection to ensure that undue external influences do not undermine their ability to give free consent.

In the United States, drawing on Nuremberg and Helsinki, the principle of informed consent was a centerpiece of the landmark *Belmont Report*, commissioned by the U.S. federal government in the 1970s. The principle was then codified under the U.S. Code of Federal Regulations in the "Common Rule," the law governing human-subjects research in the United States. This report resulted in the creation of Institutional Review Boards (IRBs) at all research institutions to oversee human-subjects research and ensure proper informed consent.

Although it began as a principle governing research on human subjects, informed consent also became a central principle of clinical ethics and the practice of medicine in the second half of the twentieth century.

Today, all fifty states have laws requiring informed consent for the prescription of medications, for diagnostic tests, and for all medical and surgical interventions—with rare exceptions only for emergency situations where consent cannot be obtained and life or limb is imminently in peril. For those lacking the capacity to consent, this still needs to be obtained with a proxy, for example, a parent, guardian, next of kin, or a conservator appointed by the court. Ethics committees have been established at all hospitals to deal with complex questions about informed consent in difficult cases. I chaired the hospital's ethics committee at the University of California, Irvine, from 2008 to 2021, where I consulted on thousands of cases involving subtleties of informed consent and decisional capacity.

● ● ●

Fast forward to 2020. During the covid pandemic, the public health and medical establishment once again abandoned the principle of free and informed consent to advance a supposed greater good. Vaccine mandates, for example, forced individuals to take products authorized only for emergency use, and thus still experimental by our own federal government's definition. Those claiming that these novel genetic therapies were no longer experimental because they had been given to millions of people only confirmed that this ongoing medical experiment was an enormous one. Under public and private employer mandates, hundreds of thousands of people lost their jobs for refusing to relinquish the right of informed consent enshrined at Nuremberg.

Under a declared state of emergency—the threshold for which our regulatory agencies deliberately never defined—the governing powers forced us to embrace a utilitarian ethic that jettisoned informed consent in the name of population health. Our leaders convinced us that the health of the social organism required this—though without a clearly defined goal for population health. We readily embraced emergency ethical standards designed to govern disaster triage, even under non-triage conditions. These crisis standards continue to dominate global health policy three years later, long after any plausible justification for sustaining an ongoing state of emergency.

Not even the obvious failure of these policies to achieve their stated aims—that is, to slow or stop the spread of the virus—proved sufficient to halt the coercive measures. Furthermore, in the few time-limited and regionally limited hotspots where covid cases approached triage conditions, almost nothing was done to alleviate this. Public health emergency plans failed to distribute health care capacity where it was most needed, which suggests that appeals to population health functioned as a pretense. In New York City, for example, overwhelmed community hospitals like Elmhurst became hotspots for covid patients to die while nearby hospitals had hundreds of empty beds.

How and why was informed consent, the bulwark of twentieth-century medical ethics, so hastily abandoned, with so little debate and almost no opposition from the medical and scientific establishments? The same cold utilitarian ethos—the ideology that governed science, medicine, and public health during the eugenics movement of the previous century—resurfaced in our day. Our public health agencies willingly embraced it, heedless of the consequences. The unholy alliance of (1) public health, (2) digital technologies of surveillance and control, and (3) the police powers of the state—what I call the Biomedical Security State—has arrived. As we will see, this biosecurity and surveillance paradigm was not created entirely de novo during the pandemic but has been in development for at least twenty years. As this book will explain, our covid policies represented only the beginning of the societal changes to come in The New Abnormal.

I'll mention here just one example of the future we can anticipate under this regime (we will see more examples in chapter 3 and the epilogue). For two decades scientists have been quietly developing self-spreading contagious vaccines.[13] The NIH (National Institutes of Health) funded this research, in which either DNA from a deadly pathogen is packaged in a contagious but less harmful virus, or the deadly virus's lethality is weakened by engineering it in a lab. The resultant "vaccines" spread from one person to the next just like a contagious respiratory virus. With this technology, only 5 percent of regional populations would need to be immunized; the other 95 percent would "catch" the vaccine as it spread person-to-person through community transmission.[14]

This technology bypasses the inconvenience of recalcitrant citizens who may refuse to give consent. Its advocates point out that a mass vaccination campaign that would ordinarily take months of expensive effort to immunize everyone could be shortened to only a few weeks. Scientists have already shown proof of concept in animal populations: In 2000, researchers in Spain tackled a deadly virus among rabbits by injecting seventy with a transmissible vaccine and returning them to the wild, where they quickly passed it on to hundreds more, thereby halting the outbreak. European countries are now testing the technology on pigs.[15]

In the wake of the covid pandemic, about a dozen research institutions in the United States, Europe, and Australia are investigating the potential human uses for self-spreading vaccines. The federal Defense Advanced Research Projects Agency (DARPA), for example, is examining this technology for the U.S. military to protect our soldiers against the West Africa Lassa fever, a virus spread from rats to humans. This project, it should be noted, does not require the consent of our military service men and women.

In 2019 the UK government began exploring this technology to address the seasonal flu. A research paper from Britain's Department of Health and Social Care advised that university students could be an obvious target group: "They do not work so [vaccinating them] will not cause much economic disruption and most have second homes to go to, thereby spreading the vaccine." Researchers admitted a contagious vaccine for an attenuated flu virus would cause some deaths but estimated these would be less than the influenza virus. As the UK government report described, "Self-spreading vaccines are less lethal but not non-lethal: they can still kill. Some people will die who would otherwise have lived, though fewer people die overall."[16] As the cynical saying goes, you can't make an omelet without breaking a few eggs. Contagious vaccines are in our future, their champions claim, and are no different than putting fluoride in drinking water. Plus, for those who find jabs unpleasant, there are fewer needles required.

Government-funded research of lab-engineered viruses to create contagious, self-spreading vaccines that bypass the consent of citizens. What could go wrong?

Well, a lot it turns out. This book is about where we are now and where the biomedical security state will lead us if we do not quickly change course. I will explore the origin and effects of novel biomedical technologies and public policy changes that accelerated during the covid pandemic, examining the militarization of public health and the associated biosecurity model of governance. We will uncover the real origins of lockdown orders, vaccine mandates and passports, and other extreme pandemic measures issued under a declared state of emergency.

While these policies were neither prudent nor scientifically sound, neither neutral nor objective, our leaders and the regulatory agencies under their purview did not enact these measures by mistake. The design, implementation, and effects of these policies were deliberately coordinated from the outset. Except for the possible release of the virus from a lab in Wuhan (which may have been unintentional), nothing during the covid pandemic happened by accident.

I write not as a detached observer, but as a physician and medical ethicist who has been deeply engaged in public policy battles from the first days of the pandemic. In 2021 I found myself in the teeth of the unfolding biomedical security regime. As I will explain in the second chapter, I sacrificed my career as an academic physician to challenge the constitutionality of vaccine mandates. This book draws upon not only my ethics and public policy research, but on my work as a physician and patient advocate over the past three years. This work took me from the frontlines of the hospital wards and medical clinics treating patients, many of whom were infected with covid and some of whom died, to the halls of power in Congress and the federal courts—where I have been battling the University of California, the CDC, the FDA, and the Biden administration on pandemic measures, data transparency, and censorship in science and public policy.

The biomedical security state has encountered pockets of resistance, though not yet enough. A developing grassroots alliance of dedicated physicians, independent journalists, self-sacrificing lawyers, and engaged citizens on every continent is mobilizing to establish resilient communities capable of exposing the problems and preventing further infiltration of our governing institutions. While "inevitablism" and fatalism are central features of The New Abnormal ideology, we can overcome these through hope, collective efforts, and solidarity. My concluding chapter explains how we can meaningfully resist the biomedical security state's new tools of intrusive surveillance and authoritarian social control, so that we may regain our freedoms and flourish together in a more rooted human future.

CHAPTER 1

Locked Up: The Biomedical Security State

People have become so used to living in a state of perennial crisis and emergency that they seem not to realize that their lives have been reduced to a purely biological state. Life is losing not only its social and political dimensions, but also its human and affective ones. A society which exists in a constant state of emergency cannot be free.

—*Giorgio Agamben*, Where Are We Now?

A new form of grassroots, working-class political engagement emerged in early 2022. When this manifestation of the medical freedom movement began in Canada, it terrified our leadership class, who were initially caught unawares. Long-haul truckers in Canada formed a convoy many kilometers long, drove together to the capital city of Ottawa, and parked their trucks downtown for an extended stay. This innovative form of protest initially arose in response to the requirement of vaccine passports at the U.S.-Canada border, a mandate instituted by Prime Minister Justin Trudeau. Instead of meeting with the truckers to discuss their concerns, Trudeau fled his capital city like a spooked child.

Trucker convoys in other countries, including the United States, followed suit. In February 2022, I found myself on Zoom calls with the organizers of the People's Convoy in the United States, which traveled from California to Washington, D.C., and back to California, where the truckers joined our second "Defeat the Mandates" march in Los Angeles in April 2022. I was happy to share the stage there with the U.S. convoy leaders. They were an example of what Edmund Burke dubbed "little platoons": self-organizing groups of ordinary citizens—the kind of initiatives that Tocqueville held up as examples of American civic engagement at its best. Both the truckers and the doctors speaking at the march were advocating for an end to the state of emergency and the cessation of covid mandates—two key elements of the emerging biomedical security state.

The Canadian truckers' protest and the U.S. convoy that followed were entirely peaceful: remarkably, they continued for weeks without a single violent incident. That is, until Canadian police roughed up some of the truckers in Ottawa when Trudeau sent in his shock troops to force the truckers out of the city. Until then the Canadian protest featured thousands of other ordinary citizens holding hands, dancing on the sidewalks, singing and playing street hockey, while kids tumbled in bouncy houses and parents lounged in hot tubs. Did it sometimes look like a gigantic block party, as critics maintained? Perhaps, but at least this was a group of citizens trying to celebrate something together in solidarity, exercising their rights to freedom of assembly and freedom of speech. It was clearly a needed reprieve from the civic wasteland of lockdowns.

The lively and playful scenes, which made the rounds on social media, suggested that after months of forced isolation, Canadians were ready to spend time with one another, even outdoors in frigid subzero temperatures. This was not exactly the makings of a seditious overthrow. Nevertheless, corporatist and statist Canadian media labored for weeks to vilify the truckers, slandering them as neo-Nazis at worst and the unwashed refuse of society at best. The reality on the ground belied these libelous smears. Even as authoritarian police confiscated fuel that the truckers were using to stay warm at night, the protestors' responses remained uniformly nonviolent. The protestors and their allies showed exceptional fortitude and restraint in response to the massive state and corporate powers arrayed against them.

Unwilling to face the truckers himself and meet with his own aggrieved citizens, Prime Minister Trudeau invoked the Emergency Act for the first time in Canadian history. Armed thereby with unprecedented powers, he sent in police to forcibly remove the truckers from the city. In a move of astonishing hubris and overweening authoritarian control, without a court order Trudeau also froze the bank accounts of the protestors, and even of Canadians who donated money to the convoy.[1] Private banking and investment firms complied with this directive, not grudgingly but eagerly, turning on their own clients to do the government's bidding and rid society of these unclean elements.[2] Imagine giving fifty dollars to support the convoy one day and going to the ATM the next, only to find that you cannot withdraw money from your bank account.

The Canadian Civil Liberties Association (CCLA) responded that "the federal government has not met the threshold necessary to invoke the Emergencies Act. This law creates a high and clear standard for good reason: the Act allows government to bypass ordinary democratic processes. This standard has not been met." They went on to explain, citing the language in the law, that the Emergencies Act can only be invoked when a situation "seriously threatens the ability of the Government of Canada to preserve the sovereignty, security and territorial integrity of Canada" and when the situation "cannot be effectively dealt with under any other law of Canada." The CCLA rightly pointed out that "governments regularly deal with difficult situations, and do so using powers granted to them by democratically elected representatives." They concluded on this cautionary note: "Emergency legislation should not be normalized. It threatens our democracy and our civil liberties."[3]

Trudeau's regime ignored these objections. Instead, it flexed its authoritarian muscle again by arresting the convoy organizers and refusing to release them on bail. Commenting on this episode, Canadian theologian Douglas Farrow wrote:

> In Ottawa . . . the public was deemed safe only if Tamara Lich, a Freedom Convoy organizer who had been denied bail, was brought into court wearing ankle cuffs. The judge ordered their removal, but the Canadian equivalent of the Committee on Public Safety had made its point: Resistance is forbidden.

Resisters will be rounded up. Their assets will be confiscated. The gulag awaits.[4]

Meanwhile, in the United States, the same week I was having a Zoom call with the organizers of the American truckers' People's Convoy, the federal Department of Homeland Security (DHS) issued a bulletin warning of anti-mandate online voices and public gatherings. The feds had apparently caught wind of the truckers' plan for a convoy from California to D.C. and were terrified that they might lose control of the pandemic narrative. According to the DHS bulletin, those who spread what the government considered "misinformation" about the pandemic, thereby undermining public trust in the U.S. government, should be considered "domestic terrorist" threats.

The message again was clear: if you challenge the government's preferred pandemic policies—including by exercising your First Amendment rights of freedom of speech and freedom of assembly, by speaking out or protesting mandates—you could be considered by Homeland Security to be, in their words, a "domestic threat actor" or a "primary terrorism-related threat," someone who is fueled by "domestic grievances often cultivated through the consumption of certain online content." Notice that Homeland Security characterized claims as "false or misleading" not when they contradict empirical evidence or scientific findings, but when they "undermine public trust in U.S. government institutions."[5]

The bulletin ignored the inconvenient fact that trust in our governing institutions had been undermined above all by the harmful pandemic policies these institutions enacted, and by their manipulative public messaging, which we will explore in the next chapter. According to the Department of Homeland Security—a federal department that did not exist twenty years ago but today has a budget of $52 billion annually—the real problem was with anyone who criticizes these policies online or in public gatherings.

In this document vigorous censorship and coordinated suppression of dissent by the federal government reached the point of accusing detractors of fomenting domestic terrorism. Lest you wonder how seriously the

DHS takes this threat, in April 2022 the DHS announced that it was creating a new Disinformation Governance Board. This came just days after Elon Musk, a free speech advocate, announced he intended to purchase Twitter. Following this announcement from the DHS, Orwell's phrase "Ministry of Truth" trended on Twitter.

Nina Jankowicz was slated to be the first executive director heading the federal Disinformation Governance Board. She is the author of *How to Lose the Information War* and *How to Be a Woman Online*. When Jankowicz released a study in 2021 called "Malign Creativity: How Gender, Sex, and Lies Are Weaponized against Women Online,"[6] she commented that, in trying to identify online "disinfo" narratives, "the biggest challenge in identifying this content both for our team and for platforms is what we've dubbed 'malign creativity'—the coded language, memes, and context-based content which allow harmful posts to avoid detection."[7] In other words, stamping out disinformation is really hard because often it's so subtle and context-dependent that censors cannot easily spot it. Last year Jankowicz posted on Twitter, "And once again for the people in the back: the 'free speech vs censorship' framing is a false dichotomy."[8] Oh, okay.

Our new Ministry of Truth would be situated squarely within the governing agency that oversees domestic intelligence and law enforcement—not exactly a department known for its transparency. As one blogger with a reputation for ironic snark put it, "DHS is the land of secret courts, secret warrants, and patriot act extra-constitutional mayhem, especially once you bring in the foreign spy and security crowd by even whispering the word 'russians' especially if you append 'elections' or 'public safety' to it."[9] In the wake of the announcement, the agency received an unexpectedly heavy wave of criticism from free speech advocates. Jankowicz stood down, and the project was temporarily put on hold—not because the administration changed its mind about the merits, but simply because this was an idea whose time had not yet come. As of this writing, the project has not been shuttered but waits on the back burner for an opportune moment.

President Clinton's former chief of staff, Rahm Emanuel, borrowing a page from Saul Alinsky's *Rule for Radicals*, remarked in 2007: "You never want a serious crisis to go to waste. And what I mean by that is an opportunity to do things you could not do before."[10] During the pandemic the government managed to do many things that it could not do before. Covid proved a useful opportunity for global elites with economic and political interests, in collaboration with the intelligence community and the police powers of the state, to accelerate the acceptance of a powerful and invasive digital infrastructure of biomedical surveillance and control.

As I will explain in this book, this system is already used for tracking and surveilling ordinary citizens, with the eventual goal of directing our behavior. During the pandemic we collectively enrolled as willing participants in massive social experiments that we never would have accepted under ordinary conditions. These normalized subtle but powerful new methods of social control. The declared state of emergency was the legal mechanism used to justify authoritarian measures the public would have otherwise rejected.

State of Emergency

In the new biomedical security state, the sovereign—the locus of political authority—is the person authorized to declare the state of emergency. At the federal level, with the backing of the president, that person is now Xavier Becerra, the Secretary of the Department of Health and Human Services (HHS), which oversees the NIH, the FDA, and the CDC, among other divisions. Becerra, a lawyer and former attorney general of California, has no medical training and zero public health experience. In the state of emergency, which Becerra and President Biden renewed again in February 2022 to almost no public notice or media attention, constitutional rules are suspended. Emergency powers are delegated to governors, public health officials, administrative state bureaucrats, committees, and even CEOs and HR directors of private companies.

Every one of the invasive policies described in the next chapter—from lockdowns and school closures to mask and vaccine mandates or passports—received its supposed legal justification from the declared state of emergency. But tellingly, the threshold for what constitutes a public health emergency—how many cases, hospitalizations, deaths, et cetera—was deliberately never defined. We could doubtless debate extensively about what the metrics for such thresholds ought to be: Should an emergency be defined by threats to the health care infrastructure, by specific morbidity and mortality counts, by characteristics of the latest variant, or by some combination of these or other metrics? But open democratic debate is precisely how we should make such prudential decisions.

In the give-and-take of political compromise, we could have developed measurable criteria or meaningful benchmarks for declaring an emergency. Such criteria could be periodically modified, but legislatively rather than by the same executive whose own authority is augmented during the state of emergency. Threshold definitional criteria are necessary to tell us not only when the governing authorities are justified in declaring a state of emergency, but just as crucially, they would indicate clearly when the emergency is over. Nearly three years into the pandemic, we neither have any such criteria nor even proposals for criteria.

President Biden's letter of February 2022 renewing the state of emergency specified no end date. The only covid statistic cited to justify indefinite continuation of the declared emergency was the total number of reported covid deaths in the United States for the entire pandemic—a cumulative number that increases monthly, even after the death rate has declined significantly. By this logic, every passing month increases the justification for the emergency measures until the monthly death count reaches zero—which will never happen for an endemic virus. But one death per month, or ten, or one hundred, one thousand, or even tens of thousands, hardly constitutes a national emergency, given baseline death rates for other illnesses like influenza, cancer, or cardiac disease that are not considered emergencies. That our federal government felt no need to justify the declared state of emergency serves as a telling reminder that our laws include no threshold requirement.

Recent history provides a broader context for governing under a state of emergency. Since World War II, the "state of exception" is no longer exceptional: in both democratic Western nations and elsewhere, declared states of emergency have frequently become the norm, continuing in some countries for decades.[11] In 1978 approximately thirty countries were operating under a state of emergency. This number rose to seventy countries by 1986. In response to the pandemic, 124 countries declared a state of emergency in 2020, with several more declaring emergencies in specific provinces and municipalities. Even prior to the pandemic, many nations operated under routinized, ongoing states of emergency. As of February 2020, there were thirty-two active national emergencies in the United States that had not been sundowned, the oldest dating back thirty-nine years, and each renewed by presidential administrations from both parties.[12]

Legal changes in Anglo-American nations over the past several decades paved the way for the state of exception to increasingly become the norm. As we saw during the pandemic, the state of exception is an essential tool deployed by the biomedical security state. The Italian philosopher Giorgio Agamben, who has studied the state of exception extensively, uses the term "biosecurity" to describe the government apparatus consisting of a new religion of health combined with state power and its state of exception: "an apparatus that is probably the most efficient of its kind that Western history has ever known."[13]

The UK Public Health Act of 1875 was amended in 1984 to allow authorities to quarantine citizens for unlimited durations without needing to prove that those quarantined were infected or contagious. Following legal changes in the wake of the September 11 terrorist attacks, U.S. governors can call a state of emergency at will, with resistance from citizens constituting a felony. These provisions are grounded in the novel legal doctrine, codified during the war on terror, that the protection of public health overrules any individual or privacy rights. This notion has been popularized by various civic duty campaigns, which focused first on mass vaccinations and later on mass quarantine.[14]

Following 9/11, the influential jurist Richard Posner argued, in an ethically dubious analysis, "Even torture may sometimes be justified in the struggle against terrorism, but it should not be considered *legally* justified."[15] Posner was employing here the logic of the state of exception, which is difficult to limit precisely because it sets aside legal constraint. But anyone who tortures another for political ends will naturally believe that torture in that instance is morally and politically justified—that this is an emergency in which the legal exception is warranted. It's surely a crisis of national security, after all; otherwise, why would we engage in torture? The justificatory line of reasoning easily becomes circular.

Posner argued that if the defense of our nation fails, then government cannot pursue any of its other goals—or as others have put it, "the Constitution is not a suicide pact."[16] But we can ask this: Every time we declare a state of emergency, suspend constitutional powers, and assume extralegal measures like torture, do we not we move our nation closer to failure? The fact that allowing practices like torture within our constitutional system would undermine this same system is perhaps evidence not for invoking the state of exception, but for the conclusion that we should not torture people, period.

Back in 2007 Posner argued that it's not only "defense against human enemies" that may justify states of emergency. To illustrate this, he asked us to "imagine strict quarantining and compulsory vaccination in response to a pandemic." Fifteen years later, we no longer need to imagine it: we can remember it. Our increasing reliance on declaring emergencies requires naming new enemies, both foreign and domestic.[17] It just so happens that invisible pathogens are a recurrent, ever-present enemy, always ready to strike with little warning, and thus always an available pretext to trigger the state of exception.

Biomedical security, which was previously a marginal part of political life and international relations, has assumed a central place in political strategies and calculations since the September 11 attacks. Already in 2005 the WHO grossly overpredicted that the bird flu (avian influenza) would kill between 2 and 150 million people. To prevent this impending disaster, the WHO made recommendations that no nation was prepared to accept at the time, which included the proposal of population-wide lockdowns. Bill Gates, the WHO's largest private supporter, has been warning of dire future pandemics for years.[18]

Even earlier, in 2001, Richard Hatchett, a member of the CIA who served also on George W. Bush's National Security Council, was already recommending obligatory confinement of the entire population in response to biological threats. Hatchett now directs the Coalition for Epidemic Preparedness Innovations (CEPI), an influential entity coordinating global vaccine investment in close collaboration with the pharmaceutical industry. CEPI is a brainchild of the World Economic Forum (WEF) in conjunction with the Bill & Melinda Gates Foundation, entities about which we will say more in chapter 3. Like many others today, Hatchett regards the fight against covid as a "war" analogous to the war on terror.[19]

By 2006 the emerging biosecurity paradigm was already distorting our federal funding priorities. That year, Congress allocated $120,000 to the National Institutes of Health (NIH) to fight influenza, which kills 36,000 Americans in a mild flu year. By contrast, Congress allocated to the NIH $1.76 billion for biodefense, even though the only biological attack on our soil, the anthrax outbreak in 2001, killed just five persons.[20]

Although proposals for lockdowns and other extraordinarily stringent measures were circulating by 2005, mainstream public health did not embrace the biosecurity paradigm until covid. According to this paradigm, a kind of overbearing medical terror is deemed necessary to deal with worst-case scenarios, whether for naturally occurring pandemics or biological weapons. Drawing on Patrick Zylberman's work, Agamben summarized the characteristics of the emerging biosecurity model, in which political recommendations had "three basic characteristics: 1) measures were formulated based on possible risk in a hypothetical scenario, with data presented to promote behavior permitting management of an extreme situation; 2) 'worst case' logic was adopted as a key element of political rationality; 3) a systematic organization of the entire body of citizens was required to reinforce adhesion to the institutions of government as much as possible."[21]

This precisely describes the pandemic strategy we adopted in 2020: (1) lockdowns were formulated based on discredited worst-case-scenario modeling from the Imperial College London; (2) this failed model over-predicted 2.2 million immediate deaths in the United States;[22] (3) consequently, the entire body of citizens, as a manifestation of civic spirit, gave up freedoms and rights in the name of a legal obligation of health. As Agamben explained, "The intended result [of this three-part framework] was a sort of super civic spirit, with imposed obligations presented as demonstrations of altruism. Under such control, citizens no longer have a right to health safety; instead, health is imposed on them as a legal obligation (biosecurity)."[23] With little resistance, we abandoned freedoms during lockdowns that were not relinquished even by the citizens of London during the city's bombing in World War II (London adopted curfews but never locked down). Even now, for many citizens, it seems not to matter that these impositions failed to deliver the promised public health outcomes.

The full significance of what transpired in March 2020 may have escaped our attention. Without realizing it we lived through the design and implementation of not just a novel pandemic strategy but a new political paradigm—a system far more effective at controlling the population than anything previously attempted by Western nations. Under the biosecurity model, "the total cessation of every form of political activity and social relationship [under lockdowns and social distancing became] the ultimate act of civic participation."[24] Neither the pre-war Fascist government in Italy nor the Communist states of the Soviet Union ever dreamed of implementing such restrictions. Social distancing became a new political paradigm for social interactions, "with a digital matrix replacing human interaction, which by definition from now on will be regarded as fundamentally suspicious and politically 'contagious,'" in Escobar's description.[25]

It is instructive to reflect on the chosen phrase, "social distancing," which is not a medical term but a political one. A medical or scientific model would have deployed a phrase like *physical* distancing or *personal* distancing, but not *social* distancing. The term suggests not a new model for health but for organizing society, one that limits human interactions by six feet of space and by masks that cover the face—our locus of interpersonal connection and communication. The six-foot distancing rule was supposedly premised on the spread of covid through respiratory droplets, though the practice continued long after it became clear that the virus spread through aerosolized mechanisms.

Actual contagion risk depended on the total time spent in a room with infected persons and was mitigated by opening windows and other methods of improved ventilation, not by staying six feet apart. Plastic protective barriers erected everywhere actually increased the risk of viral spread by impeding airflow. We were primed for over a decade to accept pseudoscientific practices of social distancing by our use of digital devices to limit human interactions. We routinely send a text message to colleagues three cubicles down rather than walking over to speak with them face-to-face. Social distancing was not entirely new; it was introduced in a particular cultural context.

The biomedical security paradigm, embraced during the pandemic, had other consequences. The growing trend for public health to expand its scope of concern and supposed expertise worked hand in glove with power grabs facilitated by declared emergencies. Recall, for example, that thousands of public health "experts" rushed to sign a statement declaring racism a public health emergency during the BLM protests of 2020. The state of emergency for covid supposedly required society-wide stay-at-home orders; but in this instance, another state of emergency for racism required the temporary suspension of these measures.

Notice how this reframed racism from a crisis of democracy (as in the 1965 Voting Rights Act) or a crisis of religion and morality (as in

Martin Luther King Jr.'s "Letter from a Birmingham Jail") to a public health crisis. This illustrates a feature of the biomedical security state: other kinds of problems—social, environmental, economic—are reframed as public health issues and eventually are declared public health emergencies. With public health takeovers like this, we paradoxically hamstring ordinary people's ability to address a problem like racism: the issue now requires the technocratic ministrations of so-called experts, and health experts no less. Authority to address the problem is taken from ordinary citizens and civic institutions and transferred to scientific ones.[26]

Our new biomedical security model of governance entails jumping from one declared crisis to the next, each time invoking the need for extra-legislative or extra-judicial executive powers to manage the declared emergency. In the state of exception, governors, presidents, and prime ministers arrogate extra-constitutional powers—or delegate such powers to their appointees—without appropriate checks and balances. In the United States, when the president declares a national emergency, he gains access to an additional 136 statutory emergency powers.[27] Governors likewise assume enormous powers when declaring a statewide emergency. And as human nature has shown time and again, once new powers are assumed, those in power are reluctant to relinquish them.

State-of-exception legal doctrines and declared public health emergencies cannot continue long in an open climate of scientific nuance and public debate. The medical, biological, and social sciences, at their best, highlight probabilities rather than certainties capable of sustaining ongoing emergencies. To resist the inclination toward scientific nuance, civic duty campaigns must convert "good citizens" into militants for the cause. The patriotic atmosphere created around emergency measures discourages any firm resistance or frontal opposition.[28] Governments leverage people's goodwill and civic spirit not only by emphasizing duties and obligations but requiring citizens to give *proofs* of altruism—visible signs like masks and obedience to stay-at-home orders, or publicly available proofs like vaccine passports. This is one reason that masks became a potent symbol of physical purity and civic spirit, as well as a symbol of mutual mistrust, during the pandemic.[29]

Consider the human goods we sacrificed to preserve bare biological life at all costs: friendships, holidays with family, work, visiting the sick and dying, worshipping God, and burying the dead. Physical human presence was confined to the enclosure of domestic walls, and even that was discouraged. Recall state governors and our president attempting to prohibit or discourage family Thanksgiving gatherings. In those dizzying early days of 2020, we lived through the swift and sustained abolition of public spaces and the squeezing even of private ones. Ordinary human *contact*, our most basic human need, was redefined as *contagion*, a threat to our existence.

Incubators of the Revolution

To see where the biomedical security state will lead, many point to the Chinese social-credit system—and this is a useful shorthand for the dystopian future this regime portends. But we need to look no further than our own American universities, which served during the pandemic as ready incubators to field-test biomedical surveillance models before they are rolled out on a mass scale. We can see the basic outlines of new developments on the horizon by examining small-scale systems recently implemented close to home.

I'll begin with a system I lived under for a brief time at the University of California, Irvine (UCI), where I was a professor of psychiatry in the School of Medicine and director of the medical ethics program. Even before vaccine passports were introduced at other public venues in the United States, my university implemented a "ZotPass" system for the digital surveillance, monitoring, and control of tuition-paying students. The ZotPass was a burdensome and invasive QR-code-facilitated regime of frequent testing, daily-symptom checklists, vaccine and booster verification, and monitoring of students' every movement on campus.

Systems like this condition students on a near constant basis to accept interdicts and strictures that only three years ago would have sounded insane. Could we have imagined in 2019 having to show a QR code testifying that we had obeyed a public health order to inject a novel pharmaceutical into our body—with the concomitant release of private health information to countless strangers—just to board a plane or to enter a restaurant? Could students have previously imagined doing this just to go to the cafeteria or gym on campus, or even to enter or leave their dorm room?

UCI's biosecurity surveillance regime was not unique among college campuses. Academia served as the test case to refine the bureaucratic systems necessary for future biosecurity measures. The political rhetoric suggested that mass vaccination in 2021 promised a return to normalcy; but what we got on campuses was not the old normal. Instead, we got the ZotPass and similar regimes at leading colleges nationwide.

For example, in September 2021, after nearly 100 percent of students, faculty, and staff had been vaccinated, Columbia University introduced new measures prohibiting students from hosting guests, visiting other residence halls, and gathering with more than ten people. Administrators had already compulsorily seized contact tracing data from students and from this data determined that a rise in cases resulted from "students socializing unmasked at gatherings in residence halls and at off-campus apartments, bars, and restaurants."[30] Imagine that—college students hanging out in dorms, bars, and restaurants.

Journalist Michael Tracey surmised that "the new powers conferred by this infrastructure—the ability to micromanage the private lives of young adults, track and adjudicate the propriety of their movements, etc.—is probably creepily intoxicating on a level these administrators may not be overtly conscious of, and in any event would almost certainly never publicly admit."[31] Though it's tempting to opine as a psychiatrist here, I will refrain from speculating on administrators' psychological motivations. What's important for our purposes is to appreciate the finely granular and intrusive level at which this invasive regime functioned.

Campus biomedical security systems relied upon an all-consuming system of thought and practice. For university administrators to wind back this regime would require an enormous psychological effort—the dismantling of a comprehensive and self-sustaining system of beliefs and regulations. Here's how Tracey describes that system:

> Benign instances of transmission—i.e., transmission that results in no severe disease, which is almost invariably the case with vaccinated young adults at astronomically low risk from COVID—would have to stop being portrayed as alarming "outbreaks," necessitating a never-ending stream of frenzied Zoom strategy meetings and swift, all-hands-on-decks interventionist tactics. The very word *outbreak* would also probably have to be ditched, given its alarmist connotations. I would suggest instead that *outbreak* be applied to these frantic upswells of bureaucratic overreaction. Perhaps the epidemiological origins of this diseased mentality could be "contact traced."[32]

Benign "cases," that is, positive PCR tests, would not have been detected if not for the compulsory and constant asymptomatic surveillance testing students were subjected to. After being conditioned with repeated covid testing, few people today can appreciate that indiscriminate asymptomatic testing violates sound principles of medical practice, creating more unnecessary problems than it solves. This principle was drilled into us in medical school; then, against all reason, it was promptly abandoned by the medical profession during covid. A "combination of bureaucratic inertia and weirdly flamboyant zeal," in Tracey's phrasing, made it hard for universities to unwind their self-perpetuating regime, even after other institutions had abandoned positive PCR tests as a useful metric.[33]

University biomedical security systems were also sustained by a near constant stream of propaganda generated by administrators, with catchphrases that would make even bureaucrats at Orwell's Ministry of Truth cringe. For example, administrators constantly admonished students, faculty, and staff to "hold one another accountable." By this they meant that students should inform on one another. You would be reported by fellow students for not wearing masks in a dorm room. You would be admonished by fellow students on the quad if your mask slipped below your nose. A student at the University of Chicago told me that all students there had to sign a Soviet-style affidavit pledging that they would snitch on fellow students for even minor violations of covid protocols.

The administrators' orders, Tracey writes, "are often cloyingly filled with artificial appeals to 'the community,' which raises the question of who elected these surveillers and snoops to be spokespersons for 'the community,' and how they even define 'communities,' which seem to contain growing segments of unwilling inhabitants."[34] Students interacting almost entirely over Zoom while isolated in dorm rooms hardly constitutes a community. As in all bureaucracies—characterized by enormous power with no locus of responsibility—such phrases also serve to deflect responsibility away from administrators for their arbitrary, invasive, and capricious rules and regulations.

Consider also that epidemiologists and infectious disease specialists were not typically drafting these university protocols. No matter how much these administrators touted their consultation with "experts," the policies were written, promulgated, and enforced by people with titles like "Associate Dean of Undergraduate Student Life" or "Assistant Dean of Institutional Equity and Inclusion." As Tracey observed, "The day-to-day decisions about practical implementation at these places often come down to the individual discretion of officials who *in no sane world* would ever be deferred to on questions of infectious disease protocol, or really anything else of significance."[35] The constant public appeal to experts masked the absence of actual expertise on the ground, giving cover for the ascent of petty tyrants.

At Georgetown the dean instructed the "Georgetown law community," 98 percent of which was vaccinated, that students in class were not allowed to remove their masks even momentarily to ask questions or drink water. After deflecting responsibility for this pronouncement by saying, "we're all in this together" and "this is your community," he encouraged students to inform on comrades who did not have a mask over both their nose and mouth by reporting this breach to the administration.[36] All for the sake of community and togetherness, of course.

His counterpart, the dean of the USC Law School, likewise sent a missive to students urging them to confront and report fellow students who were noncompliant with covid restrictions, including those who briefly lowered their mask to "hydrate." Exceptions to this rule, the dean clarified, are "limited to instructors, who may briefly hydrate while teaching but must re-mask immediately." He sternly warned that repeat violators could be subject to sanctions.[37] Law students—our country's future lawyers and politicians—were punished for hydrating, otherwise known as taking a sip of water.

We may be tempted to dismiss these regimes as so much overblown campus silliness, long characteristic of the culture of academia, in which the political battles are so fierce because the stakes are so low. But there is more happening in these cases than the latest iteration of vanguard progressivism on university campuses. We can discern here a clear sign of just how invasive, how micro, how subtly specified and overdetermined the biomedical security regime's machinations will become. Ever escalating and rigorously enforced directives will intercalate themselves into every nook and cranny of our bodily and social existence.

The UCI ZotPass and similar campus biosecurity regimes were novel social experiments, and they mostly succeeded in forcing compliance. Campus denizens generally went along, however grudgingly. A few students left college, some faculty retired early, and a handful were fired for noncompliance; but most stayed and obeyed. Indeed, students continued to pay enormous sums, often accruing massive debt, for the privilege of living under such a regime. Because, as these students had been told time and again, a university education was the only path to happiness and success.

The Megamachine

Not far from home we find another incubator of the biosecurity revolution hiding in plain sight. We just saw how the regime operates in schools; this next example shows how it operates in the workplace. Rationalized and regimented management practices, pioneered by giant tech firms like Amazon, have already created some dystopian work environments where every bodily movement is monitored and controlled at each moment. As we will see, a totalizing system of workplace conditioning and control is not just coming down the pike; it is already here, at an Amazon fulfillment warehouse near you.

I am not trying to single out one company: Amazon functions simply as the canary in the coal mine—a harbinger and innovator of trends that other firms are rapidly adopting. Many in business and industry have praised Amazon's model and are following Amazon's lead. These developments will continue to spread unless this paradigm meets significant resistance. Employee dissatisfaction and talks of unionization at Amazon suggest signs of pushback, though it's far from clear that the workers there will prevail. The odds are not presently in their favor.

The *Washington Post* ran an investigative piece with the title "Amazon's Employee Surveillance Fuels Unionization Efforts: 'It's Not Prison, It's Work.'" I give the *Post* credit for publishing this, given that the paper is owned by Amazon CEO Jeff Bezos. The piece opens with an account of Courtenay Brown, thirty-one, who works in a giant refrigerated section of an Amazon Fresh warehouse in New Jersey. She logs ten-hour days directing groceries to the right delivery truck. Amazon keeps tabs on workers through the handheld scanners they use to track inventory. Brown explains that, through this device, she is constantly "measured by a metric that calculates the amount of items her team loads to trucks along with the number of people working that shift. Amazon . . . regularly presses her to move more items with fewer people."[38]

Amazon plugs its employees into a regimented efficiency algorithm called the "Associate Development and Performance Tracker" (ADAPT). Managers can see the results in real time and scrutinize employee performance on a moment-to-moment basis, and as workers scan items, this initiates employee-performance software that minutely records precisely where products are located along with the exact speed that workers are doing their jobs at each moment. Amazon's tracking systems also "measure workers' 'time off task,' those moments when employees log off their devices—turning off their scanners or stepping away from their computers—to take a bathroom break or grab lunch."

Amazon also developed software designed to maximize staffing efficiency in its facilities, calculating "the precise number of workers it needs at any given time" and squeezing every ounce of productivity out of each one. Negative incentives, such as reprimands for poor performance metrics like logging off the system too long during bathroom breaks, are not the only method of behavioral conditioning. Amazon also uses the addictive quality of gaming competition to drive a faster work pace and squeeze more efficiency out of the workers: "The company has come up with a way to 'gamify' warehouse work, rolling out video games that run on warehouse computers and pit individuals, teams or entire floors against one another in a race to pick or stow products on its shelves," the *Post* reports.

There are cameras everywhere in an Amazon warehouse. "They basically can see everything you do, and it's all to their benefit," Ms. Brown explained. "They don't value you as a human being. It's demeaning." The *Post* article went on to note that the sentiment "that Amazon's culture of surveillance constitutes inhumane working conditions . . . has become fuel for unionization efforts to organize hundreds of thousands of workers at the country's second-largest private employer."

Kelly Nantel, speaking on Amazon's behalf, argued that employee monitoring via data collection and constant surveillance, are "prudent business measures." It is instructive to notice how the following response to employee criticism from Amazon is framed in terms of the workers' *safety* and *security*—the same justifications given for the biomedical security measures deployed during the pandemic:

> "Like any business, we use technology to maintain a level of
> *security* within our operations to help keep our employees,
> buildings, and inventory *safe*—it would be irresponsible if we

didn't do so," Nantel said in an emailed statement. "It's also important to note that while the technology helps keep our employees *safe*, it also allows them to be more efficient in their jobs" [emphasis added].[39]

The nod at the end toward efficiency marks the moment when the truth slipped out. Efficiency clearly trumps the other concerns as the highest good: the entire algorithm is oriented in that direction.

Amazon considers the development of those algorithms a competitive advantage, and the company is loath to scale them back, even with talk of unionization in the air. For many of our corporate technocrats, Amazon's surveillance-and-control system is truly a marvel. The *Post* investigation reported, "The company's surveillance of workers through the devices they use has given it scads of data to figure out the pace of work it believes is both attainable and efficient, said the [former Amazon] executive, who marvels at the innovation of the system. 'Nothing like this has been done before. There is no playbook.'"[40]

While other warehouses monitor employees with cameras and require them to hit certain productivity rates, Amazon has refined this system to new levels of intrusive specificity. The finely tuned invasive tracking of bodily movements, with built-in nudges when a worker falls behind, represents a new level of invasive industrialized control over human flesh. Human variation—one worker has prostate problems, another has menstrual issues, and yet another simply has a bad day—are not considered. The human body itself becomes part of the industrial machine: it is treated as a fungible piece of hardware controlled and directed by computer software.

The Amazon warehouse example provides a glimpse of the biosecurity model applied in the context of professional work. Those governing and directing this novel paradigm are mostly the elite class of unelected but credentialed experts and managers, technocrats who move in the virtual world of screens and software while controlling the bodies of those moving in the real world of physical labor. Amazon was among the earliest companies to employ robots in its facilities, acquiring Kiva Systems for $775 million in 2012, a manufacturer of "robotic systems that move goods throughout warehouses."[41] Humans at Amazon and other tech firms now work alongside robots, and the humans are mechanized according to the same logic.

Sitting in the airport recently, I spotted a billboard advertisement that read, "You don't have a people problem. You have a 'how you're using your people' problem. Automation can solve it." The ad was sponsored by UiPath, a global software company that sells robotic process-automation software. With a play on the word robot (indicated by a robot cartoon) the ad featured the trademarked catchphrase "Reboot Work." The ad presented automation as an icon of technological enchantment, endowing the human-replacing robot with quasi-magical liberating powers. But instead of liberating us, our increased dependence on mechanized systems forces human beings to submit to the logic of technical efficiency and docile productivity.[42]

Automation operates hand in glove with the biosecurity surveillance apparatus. Lockdowns during the pandemic accelerated automation in industries beyond manufacturing and distribution, such as hospitality. Lockdowns forced the mechanization of many jobs formerly done by humans, as a 2020 headline in *The Guardian* reported, "Robots on the Rise as Americans Experience Record Job Losses amid Pandemic."[43] These changes occurred in particular social contexts that prepared the way: new technological stages commence only after cultural changes make them conceivable. Mechanization took command of our imagination before it seized the means of production.[44]

A 2020 report from the World Economic Forum predicted that by 2025 the next wave of automation, accelerated by the pandemic, will disrupt eighty-five million jobs around the world. Echoing the UiPath's "Reboot Work" slogan, the WEF proclaimed that "businesses, governments and workers must plan to work together to implement a new vision for the global workforce."[45] All this is presented with an air of inevitability, as though human choice plays no role in these historical developments.

After the coming phase of robotic automation, humans will be demoted to a status even lower than that of cogs in the machine—for the new machine will no longer require human cogs. Without people your company no longer has a "people problem," as the UiPath advertisement promises. How convenient. And as a bonus, robots are completely immune to covid and other viral threats.

On the biosecurity surveillance workplace model, employees (when they are needed) are no longer viewed as individuals, but as fungible elements of an undifferentiated mass, to be shaped by algorithms designed to maximize productivity and efficiency. A former Amazon employee pointed out that this system does not operate on a human scale or take account of human beings as distinct individuals or free personalities: "The system doesn't recognize the human part of people, like, 'I'm having a bad day,' or 'I'm having a tough time at home.'"[46] Consider the fruits of this system: "The vortex of globalization, of modernity itself, is widening and deepening daily," Paul Kingsnorth writes, "and into it all distinctions and differences are sucked, to emerge bleached, efficient and unloved on the far shore."[47]

Because it does not operate on a human scale but treats humans like robots, or like an undifferentiated mass, the system can start to break down—or rather, the human beings caught in the system's gears can break down—under its severe regimentation. Critics have noted that Amazon's use of data it extracts by surveilling employees has led to injury rates at its facilities that are higher than industry norms. Occupational Safety and Health Administration data in 2021 showed that Amazon's serious injury rates were nearly double those at warehouses run by other companies. Likewise in 2021, Washington State's Department of Labor and Industries cited Amazon for the hazardous conditions at its warehouse in DuPont, Washington, criticizing the company's employee surveillance system. According to the citation the company received, "There is a direct connection between Amazon's employee monitoring and discipline systems and workplace MSDs [musculoskeletal disorders]."[48]

In the biosecurity surveillance paradigm, the human being is reduced to bare biological life—a mere collection of muscles, tendons, ligaments, and bones—with regrettable energy and excretion requirements. In this framework, the human "machine" can be programmed to function with maximum efficiency: digital surveillance, sophisticated algorithms, and exquisitely refined behavioral conditioning turn human flesh into a productivity engine. But like machines if you overuse them, the human body can malfunction. Not to worry, the technocrats reply, we can fine-tune the algorithm to bring each body to the brink of breakdown but not tip it over. Enthusiasts claim that science and technology will solve all the problems created by the same science and technology—a dubious notion belied by historical experience.

This entire regime of efficiency-maximizing coordination of human bodies functions in the service of cheap consumer goods, ordered online with the push of a button, and delivered by drones to your door with astonishing speed. Clicking through the Amazon app, one almost forgets there are real human beings on the other end making it all happen. As we will see in the next chapter, this business model works best—its profits skyrocket—when entire populations of people are locked down and confined. More accurately, everyone is locked down except the mechanized minions shackled to their efficiency-monitoring devices and shuttling like a hive of ants through massive Amazon warehouses. On second thought, maybe they too are locked down.

Aside from rumblings about unionization, there have been sporadic, though largely symbolic, signs of resistance. Jeff Bezos, the founding CEO of Amazon who trades places with Elon Musk for the title of richest man in the world, has like Musk invested much of his wealth in his own human spaceflight startup, a company called Blue Origin. Leading up to Bezos's own personal spaceflight in 2022, an online petition circulated: "Do not allow Jeff Bezos to return to Earth." As of this writing the petition had over two hundred thousand signatures and counting.[49] Apparently, lots of folks would be happy to see Bezos stay in outer space: perhaps there are some alien species he can colonize and mechanize.

In a similar vein, *Vanity Fair* reported in 2020 that protestors demanding higher wages and decent working conditions for Amazon workers set up a guillotine outside Bezos' $23 million home (a mere 0.0115 percent of his total net worth) in Washington, D.C.[50] These protestors wondered why Amazon could spend billions on sending its founder and other billionaires to space, but could not offer its minions a decent wage, personal protective equipment, or a few more bathroom breaks. While I don't endorse their violent Jacobin symbolism—the French Revolution cannibalized itself, after all—I do sympathize with the sentiments expressed. I might, however, gently remind the protestors that the system of rationalized mass death symbolized by the guillotine is not the answer, but in fact the violent offspring of the very problem they claim to resist.[51] Even the resistance can all too easily be coopted by the machine.

● ● ●

Both the university campus and the Amazon warehouse examples demonstrate that the biomedical security paradigm is not just a prediction about what is coming, not merely a prophetic conjecture about the future, but a system that has already arrived. While the full manifestation of this regime is not yet here, many of its central features are already with us in embryonic form. Some of them, such as a willingness to hand over massive amounts of personal data for the sake of convenience, are things that most of us have grown accustomed to; these no longer give us much pause.

Over fifty years ago, Lewis Mumford foresaw these developments in his classic 2-volume study, *The Myth of the Machine*. Mumford's work described the growing technocratic power that threatened to overwhelm our humanity—what he called the megamachine. This is a machine made not of gears and pulleys, but a *machine made of human parts*. It is driven by "order, power, predictability and above all, control." With his far-seeing eye, Mumford wrote as though he had experienced a vision of a twenty-first-century Amazon warehouse situated within a network of global distribution arteries:

> With this new "megatechnics" the dominant minority will create a uniform, all-enveloping, super-planetary structure, designed for automatic operation. Instead of functioning actively as an autonomous personality, man will become a passive, purposeless, machine-conditioned animal whose proper functions, as technicians now interpret man's role, will either be fed into the machine or strictly limited and controlled for the benefit of depersonalized, collective organizations.[52]

In his commentary on this theme, Paul Kingsnorth observes that "those 'depersonalized, collective organizations' are the giant world-spanning corporations" which now dominate the landscape and exercise outsized control over our lives, our politics, and our media. He refers to the internet as the "neurological network of the Machine." Given the internet's ubiquitous presence in our lives, "there are now few places on Earth we can escape from the incessant noise of this State-corporate 'growth,' and the incessant urge to contribute to it by clicking, scrolling, buying and competing."[53]

In describing the original example of the megamachine, Mumford explained what happens to the human beings when they are reduced to parts in this rationalized system of efficiency and control:

> The workers who carried out these designs had minds of a new order: mechanically conditioned, executing each task in strict obedience to instructions, infinitely patient, limiting their response to the word of command. Machine work can be done only by machines. These workers during their period of service were, as it were, stripped down to their reflexes, in order to ensure a mechanically perfect performance.[54]

The system he is referring to in this passage is not an Amazon warehouse, or a British factory in the age of the Industrial Revolution, but a much older system. The original megamachine—the paradigmatic machine made of human parts—was the system that built the Egyptian pyramids. There's a reason we refer to those helpless Egyptian laborers as slaves. "The Machine is, to its core," Kingsnorth writes, "anti-limits and anti-form: which means anti-nature, and thus anti-human."[55] As Mumford warned us a half-century ago, the megamachine ultimately leads to violence, despotism, and death.

Our Digital Panopticon

The biomedical security state requires the power to monitor and control the movements and behaviors of an entire population, understood as a vector of disease, to manage a microbial threat. This requires surveillance capacities made possible only by digital technologies. Given that the iPhone was released in 2007, it is no coincidence that the emergence of the biomedical security paradigm coincided with the advent of digital technologies capable of tracking citizens movements at every moment and data mining their private communications and market exchanges.

In November 2021 Israel passed emergency pandemic legislation that permitted the Shin Bet, the nation's equivalent of the CIA, to access mobile phones and extract track and trace data from suspected omicron patients without their consent. The *New York Times* quoted Limor Yehuda, a criminology professor supportive of this move, who remarked: "We have indeed reached a point at which we do need a 'Big Brother' keeping track of where we go." He argued that this level of surveillance was necessary to quickly identify potential virus carriers who need to be tested and quarantined.

The *Times* also reported that pre-pandemic war-gaming exercises influenced Israel's unprecedented actions during the pandemic:

In that exercise, senior officials simulated how they would respond to a fictional scenario that bore striking similarities to what is actually happening now. . . . In the simulation, officials . . . decided to keep Israel's borders open to tourists into December, only to find that by the later stages of the exercise, the country's hospitals were overwhelmed with patients. The correct decision, the participants concluded afterward, would have been to close Israel's borders to most foreigners immediately, according to Yaacov Ayish, a retired general who helped plan the drill. "It was one of the lessons," Mr. Ayish said. "Suddenly, all the government agencies and the military had to analyze it as an option."[56]

We see in Israel's response to the omicron variant all three basic characteristics of the biosecurity paradigm described earlier. First, measures are formulated based on possible risk in a hypothetical scenario, with data presented to promote behavior permitting management of an extreme situation. Typically, viruses tend to evolve by becoming more contagious but less deadly. This is because a virus "wants" to propagate but cannot do so if it kills too many hosts. It was therefore foreseeable that omicron would be less lethal than delta, yet Israel's war-game scenario predicted that hospitals would be overwhelmed with cases from a new variant. This illustrates the second feature of the biosecurity paradigm: "worst case" logic is adopted as a key element of political rationality.

The third feature suggests that a systematic organization of the entire body of citizens is required to reinforce adhesion to the institutions of government as much as possible. When the real omicron variant arrived, based on the biosecurity logic developed in Israel's recent pandemic war-game simulation, Israeli legislators decided it was necessary to have their intelligence agency spy on their own citizens. This authoritarian invasion of privacy was done not because ordinary citizens were suspected of domestic terrorism, but because they might have been in contact with someone who had a virus that caused common-cold symptoms in almost all infected individuals.

Israel was not alone in this. In October 2021 the former privacy commissioner of Ontario, Ann Cavoukian, expressed concern that Canada's vaccine passport system would amount to an intrusive surveillance regime that requires citizens to reveal private health information and tracks their movements. Two months later, Canada's Public Health Agency confirmed it had indeed been tracking mobile phone data from the outset of the pandemic, covertly analyzing citizens' movements to inform its pandemic response. The agency also revealed that it planned on expanding the program to other health issues and continuing it until 2026. Prime Minister Trudeau had previously disavowed this strategy publicly back in March 2020. But his government did it nevertheless, without public notification or consent.[57]

In May of 2022, *Vice* broke the story that during the previous two years the "CDC tracked millions of phones to see if Americans followed COVID lockdown orders." According to documents obtained by Motherboard, the CDC used "phone location data to monitor schools and churches" and planned to also use the data for applications beyond covid: "The documents also show that although the CDC used COVID-19 as a reason to buy access to the data more quickly, it intended to use it for more-general CDC purposes." The recovered CDC documents, dating from 2021, state that the data "has been critical for ongoing response efforts, such as hourly monitoring of activity in curfew zones or detailed counts of visits to participating pharmacies for vaccine monitoring."

"The documents contain a long list of what the CDC describes as 21 different 'potential CDC use cases for the data.'" These include, among other applications, monitoring curfews, neighbor-to-neighbor visits, visits to churches and other places of worship, school visits, and "examination of the effectiveness of public policy on [the] Navajo Nation." Other uses mentioned include public health issues besides covid, such as "research points of interest for physical activity and chronic disease prevention such as visits to parks, gyms, or weight management businesses," as well as "exposure to certain building types, urban areas, and violence."

Although the data purchased by the CDC was aggregated to show trends, "researchers have repeatedly raised concerns with how location data can be deanonymized and used to track specific people."[58] Research has demonstrated that unmasking specific users from these aggregated mobility datasets is quite feasible. One research team, for example, studied fifteen months of human mobility data for one and a half million individuals and published their results in *Nature*: "In a dataset where the location of an individual is specified hourly and with a spatial resolution equal to that given by the [mobile phone] carrier's antennas, four spatio-temporal [data] points are enough to uniquely identify 95% of the individuals." The researchers coarsened the spatio-temporal data and still found "even coarse datasets provide little anonymity."[59]

The CDC purchased its data from the controversial broker SafeGraph, a company that, according to CDC documents, offers data that "allows for extremely accurate insights related to age, gender, race, citizenship status, income, and more." Due to its questionable practices, SafeGraph was banned from the Google Play Store in June 2021, which meant that "any app developers using SafeGraph's code had to remove it from their apps." The company includes among its key investors the former head of Saudi intelligence. This is where the CDC went to get its tracking data, paying SafeGraph $420,000 for access to one year of data.[60]

Evidence also emerged recently that the CIA has been using unauthorized digital surveillance to spy on Americans. After supporting vaccine mandates in 2021, the ACLU finally took an interest again in civil liberties in 2022. They expressed alarm when newly declassified documents revealed that the CIA has been secretly conducting massive surveillance programs that capture Americans' private information. Like the Shin Bet in Israel, our federal intelligence agency has been spying not on suspected terrorists but on ordinary Americans, with no judicial oversight and without congressional approval.

As the ACLU noted, "This surveillance is done without any court approval, and with few, if any, safeguards imposed by Congress to protect our civil liberties." They argued: "These reports raise serious questions about what information of ours the CIA is vacuuming up in bulk and how the agency exploits that information to spy on Americans. This invasion of our privacy must stop."[61] Though the ACLU arrived a bit late to the party, as the old saying goes, better late than never.

U.S. senators Ron Wyden of Oregon, and Martin Heinrich of New Mexico, both Democrats and members of the Senate Intelligence Committee, called for the declassification and investigation of relevant CIA documents. In a letter of April 13, 2021, which they made public, the two senators expressed concern that the CIA program was "entirely outside the statutory framework that Congress and the public believe govern this collection [of data], and without any of the judicial, congressional or even executive branch oversight that comes from [Foreign Intelligence Surveillance Act—FISA] collection." Despite Congress's clear intent, with the support of the American people, to limit warrantless collection of Americans' private records, the senators warn, "these documents reveal serious problems associated with warrantless backdoor searches of Americans, the same issue that has generated bipartisan concern in the FISA context."[62]

There is a broader legal context for these extra-legal developments of mass surveillance of civilian populations. Since the war on terror began, Western nations have legislatively scaled up their increasingly intrusive networks of mass surveillance—often referred to with the euphemism "bulk collection." The last decade has seen such measures passed in the United Kingdom, France, Australia, India, Sweden, and other countries—not to mention the AI-enabled facial- and gate-recognition surveillance in China, technology that Xi Jinping is already exporting to eager rogue regimes around the globe.[63]

In the United States, even if Congress manages to rein in what appears to be the CIA's extra-judicial activities—and we must hope that they do—this alone will not solve our surveillance problems. For in the contemporary context, mass surveillance can be conveniently crowd-sourced. Social media groupthink and scapegoating enable citizens to surveil and punish one another in online environments. In *The Crowd-Sourced Panopticon: Conformity and Control on Social Media*, Jeremy Weissman makes the case that Twitter and other online platforms function in precisely this way.

Twitter mobs are a powerful social force that ideologues can manipulate to their advantage, particularly when Twitter and Facebook can put their thumbs on the scale by tweaking their algorithms. Some of us worry about government eavesdropping and corporate data harvesting; but in a more tangible way, most of us fear the public eye and its tools of social and professional censure. The societal effects of this may be far more consequential than anything dreamed up by CIA or NSA spooks.

The implicit threat of cancellation or online public humiliation enforces tight social conformity. Online carrots and sticks can turn us into a kind of "personality machine," in Weissman's phrase, "emptied out and programmed by society, watching oneself do as society signals one to do." In this digital environment, we "judge ourselves based on how others judge us on the screen, and act out the desired roles as directed accordingly." The willingness of people to cancel relationships with friends and family over political differences or different views of covid policies suggests the strength of these performative roles in shaping our identity. As many of us experienced in the last few years, while these tendencies have been developing for a decade, they accelerated dramatically during the pandemic.[64]

● ● ●

Jeremy Bentham was an eighteenth-century philosopher and social reformer. Along with John Stuart Mill, Bentham is best known as one of the philosophical advocates of utilitarianism, the ethical theory that the ends do justify the means, so long as we aim at "the greatest happiness for the greatest number." We can do bad things (for example, lie, steal, and cheat) if the overall outcomes result in an increase of overall happiness. This philosophy amounts to a kind of superstition according to which, by some mysterious mechanism, the deployment of sheer force automatically produces justice. Utilitarian "ethics" enjoyed a boon during the pandemic, but one of Bentham's other contributions is even more relevant to our present moment.

Bentham pioneered what he called a "panopticon," a blueprint for a system of surveilling and completely controlling a population. The floor plan involved a circular building with a guard at the center who could observe around the clock all the surrounding cells along the periphery. Although the design suggests a prison, Bentham maintained that the panopticon was "a new principle of construction applicable to any sort of establishment, in which persons of any description are to be kept under inspection." Besides prisons, he also suggested its use in quarantine stations, poorhouses, houses of industry, factories, hospitals, workhouses, madhouses, and alas, schools.[65]

The panopticon's principle of radical transparency promised to rationalize the discipline of otherwise unruly populations. Because individuals could be observed at any moment, whether they were in fact observed or not, they would remain constantly on guard. Denizens inside the panopticon would self-police their behaviors and internalize the mechanisms of control. Through constant fear of punishment, prisoners would learn to patrol themselves. George Orwell captured this in his dystopian novel, *Nineteen Eighty-Four*, with his description of Big Brother's ubiquitous television screens with built-in cameras, always on and always watching you: "You had to live—did live, from habit that became instinct—in the assumption that every sound you made was overheard, and, except in darkness, every movement scrutinized."[66]

The French philosopher Michel Foucault argued that the panopticon is not primarily a design for a building, but a metaphor for the exercise of political power in modern societies. In 1975 Foucault gave the following description in *Discipline and Punish*: "The Panopticon must not be understood as a dream building: it is the diagram of a mechanism of power reduced to its ideal form." He goes on to explain, "It is in fact a figure of political technology that may and must be detached from any specific use."[67]

With the advent of technologies of mass surveillance, we now live in a kind of worldwide digital panopticon, where each citizen is simultaneously guard and fellow prisoner. In totalitarian societies one does not just fear the censure of the ruler, one fears everyone else, for every neighbor is a potential informant. Today, every potential informant is armed with a smartphone camera in his pocket. This means that the digital panopticon is more than just a metaphor: real people really are watching. Recall how university administrators encouraged students to act as informants during covid to enforce strict compliance with the minutiae of their covid protocols.

The power of our contemporary peer-to-peer crowdsourced panopticon is enhanced by novel technologies. Ray-Ban's "smart glasses," modeled on the Google Glass prototype, threaten to make invisible cameras omnipresent. The digital panopticon's "data is stored online, almost never disappears, and is easily searchable. Information crosses the globe in the blink of an eye. The Stasi and KGB could only have dreamed of such a system."[68]

During the pandemic we reached a level of detailed behavioral scrutiny and social control—"pull your mask up over your nose"—never previously encountered in public social settings. Nobody wants to live in a house made entirely of glass with no way to pull down the shades. While a worldwide panopticon sounds to most people like a dystopian nightmare, many of our ruling technocrats hope to soon produce just such a society. For example, "former Google CEO Eric Schmidt dreams of a world where 'everything is available, knowable, and recorded by everyone all the time.'" Meanwhile, "Airbnb founder Brian Chesky believes that a digitally enabled 'reputation economy' [that is, a social-credit system] will allow for 'so many different activities that we can't even imagine right now.'" As Professor Taylor Dotson shrewdly observed, "a radically transparent society also conveniently aligns with Silicon Valley's dominant business model."[69]

The global digital panopticon discourages passionate commitments and encourages not just conformity, but a kind of conformity that's easily manipulated by mass media or economic conglomerates. Don't take risks, just pull that mask up and sanitize your hands again. If you refuse to comply, the consequences could be serious. We'll look at just one example of the digital panopticon's operation during the pandemic. A 2020 *New Yorker* essay told the story of Dr. Wojciech Rokita, a gynecologist and obstetrician in Poland, who served as a regional governmental health consultant during the pandemic.

Dr. Rokita had made significant contributions to public health during his career. Under his direction, the region's neonatal mortality rate improved dramatically. In 2018, at the age of fifty-two, "his peers elected him head of the Polish Society of Gynecologists and Obstetricians." In March 2020 before Poland had any confirmed covid cases, Dr. Rokita and his wife traveled to the Swiss Alps for a ski vacation. Worried about a new covid outbreak in Switzerland, he headed home early and got tested. Poland shut its borders three days after he arrived home, but he tested positive.

A tabloid called *Echo Dnia* reported that the first patient in the region to test positive was a local doctor. Within a half hour of the article appearing online, Dr. Rokita was revealed in the comments section of the article. The storm of public vitriol commenced immediately: outraged comments flooded in, including from people who knew him personally, as the *New Yorker* reported:

> "I'm certainly not going to let this go just because—thank God—I didn't go to my appointment," a hospital worker who was also a private patient of Rokita's wrote, anonymously. "He could have consciously and deliberately infected me." She added, "I wonder how many women weren't as lucky as I was last week." Video surveillance showed no sign of Rokita's having been at the hospital before he started quarantining there. . . . A commenter on the *Echo Dnia* Web site

said of Rokita, "Someone should spit in his face." Another wrote, "If he went skiing during the epidemic, and he's really a doctor, then I think he's a brainless moron."[70]

The *New Yorker* reported that "Rokita's cell phone was so overwhelmed by vitriolic calls that his family couldn't get through to him. They began to worry that someone would burn down their house." Rokita, who was quarantining in the hospital by his choice, called the newspaper and begged the paper to stop publishing the hateful comments. The editor responded that "limiting comments on the paper's Facebook page" would only increase people's anger. Rokita's daughter Karolina told a reporter, "He was overwhelmed. Not only with the amount of hate comments, messages, phone calls he was receiving—even at 4 a.m.—but also with the fact that the attack came from people he knew and had helped in the past."

A few days later, while still in the hospital, Dr. Rokita took his own life. The newspaper that had destroyed him was the first to report on his suicide, before his family was even informed. An online commentator quickly revealed that he had died by hanging. His daughter maintains his suicide was Rokita's attempt to end the attacks his family was experiencing, as she explained: "The same way we were scared for him, he was scared for us." No funeral home would accept his body. The hospital cremated his remains without the family's consent. Hospital officials insisted that his family go to "a location outside the city limits to take possession of his ashes, as if he had been a medieval leper."

Even after his death, the verbal attacks continued, with some commentators calling his suicide a "foolish overreaction."[71] Mimetic social censure and scapegoating are powerful forces, and online mob behaviors die hard.

War-Gaming Pandemics

In the last section, we saw that retired Israeli generals coordinated pandemic preparation drills, but this practice was hardly unique to

Israel. Intelligence and other government agencies in the United States, in collaboration with public and private sector interests, have likewise been war-gaming pandemic scenarios for over two decades. The merging of public health and the military-intelligence-industrial complex did not begin with covid. Public health's gradual militarization is a decades old development, massively accelerated by the covid pandemic to be sure, but prepared by over twenty years of coordinated efforts.

Following the collapse of the Soviet Union in 1989, the military-industrial complex in the United States was casting about for a new enemy to keep its machinery operating and taxpayer capital flowing. Terrorism served this purpose for about ten years after 2001, but over the past decade the industry found its foil in an old enemy that could be recast as a perennial and invisible threat: microbes—whether of natural or artificial origin. Like terrorism, viral and other microbial threats are, conveniently for those who stand to profit, an enemy that can never be fully vanquished.

In the decades before covid, public and private institutional leaders in the United States ran several dry run tabletop simulations that anticipated and prepared our disastrous covid response. In 1999 the U.S. Department of Health and Human Services, in collaboration with the newly formed Johns Hopkins Center for Civilian Biodefense Strategies (later renamed the Center for Health Security), hosted a simulation of a smallpox terrorist attack. Following the exercise, frontline medical teams recommended an increase in administrative state powers to impose quarantine, isolation, media censorship, and even the intervention of the military during a public health crisis.

Shortly afterwards U.S. lawmakers introduced these proposed recommendations, adding to them the empowering of local police and the National Guard during public health emergencies. In 2002 these were codified in federal law as the "U.S. Public Health Security & Bioterrorism Preparedness & Response Act." The new law, which permitted quarantine, isolation, and censorship, applied not only to the sick but also to asymptomatic persons. While laws of this kind remain less common in Europe, a similar law was soon instituted in France.[72]

Similar pandemic war-game scenarios continued for the next fifteen years, complete with names straight out of central casting, including Dark Winter (2001), Atlantic Storm (2003, 2005), Global Mercury (2003), Lockstep (2010), Mars (2017), SPARS (2017), Clade X (2018), and Crimson Contagion (2019). Consistent themes included militarizing medicine and empowering centralized authoritarian governance capable of broad surveillance and behavioral control of large populations. Every one of these scenarios ended with coerced mass vaccination.

Each of these exercises predicted necessary futures that most ordinary people would find dystopian, but which the participants consistently described as "the new normal." Robert F. Kennedy Jr. summarized the common elements in all these pandemic war games: "The simulations war-gamed how to use police powers to detain and quarantine citizens, how to impose martial law, how to control messaging by deploying propaganda, how to employ censorship to silence dissent, and how to mandate masks, lockdowns, and coercive vaccinations and conduct track-and-trace surveillance among potentially reluctant populations."[73] The options that these scenarios never considered were just as significant as the solutions that they examined, as Kennedy also noted:

> None of them emphasized protecting public health by showing Americans how to bolster their immune systems, to eat well, to lose weight, to exercise, to maintain vitamin D levels, and to avoid chemical exposure. None of these focused on devising the vital communications infrastructures to link frontline doctors during a pandemic or to facilitate the development and refinement of optimal treatment protocols. None of these dealt seriously with the need to identify off-the-shelf (now known as "repurposed") therapeutic drugs to mitigate fatalities and to shorten a pandemic's duration. None of them considered ways to isolate the sick and protect the vulnerable—or how to shield

people in nursing homes and other institutions from infection. None of them questioned the efficacy of masks, lockdowns, and social distancing in reducing casualties. None of them engaged in soul-searching about how to preserve constitutional rights during a global pandemic.[74]

This series of pandemic war games culminated in an astonishing simulation exercise, which preceded the first publicly reported case of covid by only a few weeks. In October 2019 the renamed Johns Hopkins Center for Health Security, in partnership with the World Economic Forum and the Bill & Melinda Gates Foundation, organized a tabletop pandemic simulation scenario with epidemiologists and other experts called "Event 201: A Global Pandemic Exercise." I recommend you watch this simulation online: the entire 4-part event and a shorter twelve-minute highlight version are available on YouTube.[75]

Participants included high-ranking individuals from the World Bank, the World Economic Forum, the Chinese government, the world's largest pharmaceutical company (Johnson & Johnson), the CDC, a former NSA/CIA director, and Avril Haynes, later tapped by Biden to be the director of national intelligence—the highest-level intelligence official in the United States. Several of the participants in this simulation quickly moved into key positions to run our real covid pandemic response only a few months later.

I'll mention a few highlights from the scripted scenario and tabletop discussion, where Bill Gates instructed participants to role-play as members of an international "Pandemic Control Council." A new coronavirus (yes, you read that right) begins in pigs and spreads to humans, causing flu-like symptoms and pneumonia. Farmers start getting sick and the virus quickly spreads to become a global pandemic, with large numbers of people requiring intensive care and many dying. "There are problems emerging that can only be solved by global business and governments working together," Tom Inglesby, director of the Johns Hopkins Center for Health Security, informs the Council.

A news anchor on the fictional "GNN" network interrupts the discussion to inform participants that scientists are not optimistic about having a vaccine ready in time. Antivirals and other medical supplies are also in short supply, the news reports. Adrian Thomas of Johnson & Johnson testifies that a "global fund" that will serve as "a centralized mechanism capable of procuring pandemic supplies" is absolutely necessary. Count on the corporate executive at the table to pitch public funding for private enterprise.

Sofia Borges of the U.N. Foundation then asserts that the United Nations, of which the WHO is a subsidiary, needs "a worldwide footprint" to help poorer countries during the pandemic. Christopher Elias from the Gates Foundation next argues that international organizations like the WHO must partner with private organizations (you might guess which ones) to facilitate an international stockpile of pandemic supplies like vaccines and "make smart decisions about how to allocate them to people who need them." Then, in astonishingly telling remarks, Jane Halton of the ANZ Bank group explains not only the need to secure payments for the necessary supplies but also the need for governments to guarantee markets for their consumption:

> So, to be completely clear, most of this production would already be completely committed in contracts. It is almost unheard of that people are producing product without having a forward commitment for the consumption of their product. So [this is] the first thing that needs to be done—because this is not something that countries control unless countries bring about emergency situations and co-opt an existing supply chain.

A note of realpolitik creeps in when Stephen Redd of the CDC worries that "countries are not going to buy countermeasures to put into a global supply without retaining a large portion of it for themselves." GNN reporters again interrupt the roundtable discussion to update participants on the state of the pandemic: countries have banned travel from the worst-affected regions, and as a result "the travel and airline sectors are taking huge economic hits" with "a ripple effect racing through the tourist sector," which eventually leads to a "growing global financial crisis." The CDC's Redd, outfitted in the uniform of a military officer, chimes in again and explains that to manage the financial crisis, "governments will need to be willing to do things that are out of their historical perspective; it's really a war footing that we need to be on."

The next GNN broadcast reports that countries are reacting in different ways regarding "how to handle dis- and mis-information" about the pandemic on the internet. "In some cases, limited internet shutdowns are being implemented to quell the panic." Lavan Thiru, a monetary authority in Singapore, speculates that governments need to step up their suppression of "fake news," and other participants opine on the need for "a technological answer to this." Matthew Harrington of Edelman, the world's leading corporate PR firm, then explains that social media companies cannot see themselves as technology platforms but as broadcasters, and "they in fact have to be a participant in broadcasting accurate information and partnering with the scientific and health communities to counterweight, if not flood the zone, of accurate information." The people sitting around the table doubtless assume they will be the ones to determine what information is accurate.

The pandemic exercise culminates in a compulsory mass vaccination campaign, during which the Council participants strategize about how to use censorship and other authoritarian measures to silence recalcitrant dissidents. Not to be outdone on this score, George Gao, director of the Chinese version of the CDC, worries about how to suppress inevitable rumors that the virus came from a lab: "People believe, 'this is a manmade [pathogen]' . . . and that some pharmaceutical company made the virus," he complains during the Council's roundtable discussion. Two months later, Gao led the Chinese efforts to discredit the covid lab-leak hypothesis. Life imitates art.

A narrator concludes Event 201 by informing us, "The outcome of [the scenario] was *catastrophic*. Sixty-five million people died in the first eighteen months." It's instructive to note the alarmist language (here italicized) she employs throughout her closing monologue: "The outbreak was small at first and initially seemed controllable" but then spread worldwide to crowded mega-cities and spread became "*explosive*." The narrator continued: "The global economy was in a *freefall*, the GDP down 11 percent, stock markets around the world *plummeted* between 20 and 40 percent and headed into a *downward cycle of fear* and low expectation," she explains. The monologue continues, "Economists say the economic *turmoil* caused by such a pandemic will last for years, perhaps a decade. The societal impacts, the loss of faith in governments, the distrust of news, and the *breakdown* of social cohesion could last even longer."

The narrator then explains that these catastrophic consequences could have been avoided with ten years of proactive pandemic planning, utilizing the strategies advocated by the participants in the war-game exercise. She closes with the question, "So, are we as a global community now finally ready to do the hard work needed to prepare for the next pandemic?"[76] Considering that Event 201 was staged a few weeks before anyone had heard of covid, but while Wuhan was simultaneously seeing its first unreported cases of the novel pathogen, we must admit that this was quite a remarkable script.

Event 201 did not arise from nowhere, as suggested by the list of previous pandemic war games given above. We'll look briefly at just one among its several precedents. Ten years prior, in 2009, President Obama declared that biosecurity was central to foreign policy in memos sent to various government agencies, which instructed them to integrate this paradigm into their mission. The following year, Bill Gates delivered his "Decade of Vaccines" speech at the United Nations. A few days after that, we got the publication of a report funded by the Rockefeller Foundation, written by Peter Schwartz, founder of the Global Business Network (GBN). The document, which carried the nondescript title *Scenarios for the Future of Technology and International Development*, contained four scenarios illustrating how its principles might be advanced. One of these scenarios was called "Lock Step."

Lock Step reinforces the idea that rigid, global, authoritarian responses are necessary for the containment of infectious diseases. It's worth noting that Schwartz, the document's author, maintained deep connections to U.S. intelligence, the oil industry, and Silicon Valley. He helped launch *Wired* magazine in 1993, which became a clearinghouse for intelligence chatter as well as tech news. The Lock Step scenario posits that in 2012, "the pandemic that the world had been anticipating for years finally hit" in the form of a new deadly and highly contagious influenza strain "originating from wild geese."

"Even the most pandemic prepared nations were quickly over-whelmed when the virus streaked around the world, infecting nearly 20 percent of the global population and killing 8 million in just seven months." The international economy grinds to a halt with global supply chains shattered. Local office buildings are abandoned.

At first, lax responses make things worse: "The United States' initial policy of 'strongly discouraging' citizens from flying proved deadly in its leniency, accelerating the spread of the virus not just within the U.S. but across borders." The United States' entire political response likewise proves ineffective. "However, a few countries did fare better—China in particular," the script explains. "The Chinese government's quick imposition and enforcement of mandatory quarantine for all citizens, as well as its instant and near-hermetic sealing off of all borders, saved millions of lives, stopping the spread of the virus far earlier than in other countries and enabling a swifter post-pandemic recovery."[77] There's a reason this scenario is entitled Lock Step.

The text displays no squeamish scruples in lauding the paradigm that ultimately prevails:

> China's government was not the only one that took extreme measures to protect its citizens from risk and exposure. During the pandemic, national leaders around the world flexed their authority and imposed airtight rules and restrictions, from the mandatory wearing of face masks to body

temperature checks at the entries to communal spaces like train stations and supermarkets. Even after the pandemic faded, this more authoritarian control and oversight of citizens and their activities stuck and even intensified. In order to protect themselves from the spread of increasingly global problems—from pandemics and transnational terrorism to environmental crises and rising poverty—leaders around the world took a firmer grip on power.[78]

The Lock Step scenario then imagines the developments in subsequent years. Initially the concept of "a more controlled world gained wide acceptance and approval. Citizens willingly gave up some of their sovereignty—and their privacy—to more paternalistic states in exchange for greater safety and stability." In fact, many embraced top-down direction: "In developed countries, this heightened oversight took many forms: biometric IDs for all citizens, for example, and tighter regulation of key industries whose stability was deemed vital to national interests." And "in many developed countries, enforced cooperation with a suite of new regulations and agreements slowly but steadily restored both order and, importantly, economic growth."

The scenario does posit some forecasted downsides: cronyism in the developing world, reactionary nationalistic movements, and some inhibition of entrepreneurial activity due to stringent industry regulations. Lock Step projects that thirteen years after the pandemic, "people seemed to be growing weary of so much top-down control and letting leaders and authorities make choices for them," resulting in "sporadic pushback" that "became increasingly organized."

"Even those who liked the greater stability and predictability of this world began to grow uncomfortable and constrained by so many tight rules and by the strictness of national boundaries. The feeling lingered that sooner or later, something would inevitably upset the neat order that the world's governments had worked so hard to establish."[79] There you have it: the main long-term worry is that this *neat order* might eventually be disrupted.

Finally, during the covid pandemic in May 2021, the Nuclear Threat Initiative (NTI) and the Munich Security Council (MSC) convened an international pandemic war game, a "tabletop exercise on reducing high-consequence biological threats." The scenario had participants imagine a "global pandemic involving an unusual strain of Monkeypox" beginning one year later, on May 15, 2022. In typical pandemic war-game style, the biosecurity simulation script imagined catastrophic outcomes with over a quarter of a billion deaths worldwide from the genetically engineered monkeypox strain.[80] Although the name sounds like it was written for a dystopian movie script, monkeypox is a virus discovered in Africa in 1958; roughly 1 percent to 3 percent of cases are fatal.

Then, in mid-May 2022, right on schedule, authorities in the real world reported outbreaks of monkeypox in Europe, the United Kingdom, the United States, and Australia. The WHO convened an emergency meeting to address the outbreak a few days later. *Fortune* magazine reported on May 19 that the "U.S. government places $119 million order for 13 million freeze-dried Monkeypox vaccines," with an option to buy another $180 million worth of vaccines from biotech company Bavarian Nordic. Technically, these were smallpox vaccines that are reported to be 85 percent effective against monkeypox.[81] This purchase seemed entirely unnecessary since we already have a supply of the smallpox vaccine in our Strategic National Stockpile (SNS) large enough to vaccinate "the entire U.S. population." The SNS also has plenty of antiviral drugs to treat smallpox infections if necessary. In July 2022 the WHO declared monkeypox a public health emergency; in August 2022 California did likewise, declaring a state of emergency after eight hundred cases were reported in the state, virtually all caused by close sexual contact among men who have sex with men.[82]

The biomedical security strategy, war-gamed in tabletop exercises and scenarios like Event 201 and Lock Step, resulted in increased legal measures authorizing enhanced policing and detention capacity. These still rely for their legitimacy, however, on the public's trust in public health authorities. Prior to covid, the United States did not have a widely recognized public health authority instantiated in a single public health officer. We saw efforts during covid to construct Anthony Fauci as just such a visible authority. Similarly, Rochelle Walensky, a previously unknown researcher appointed as the CDC director during the pandemic, was often framed as a visible locus of authority.

As an aside, while we were both presenting on a covid panel to legislators from various European countries, the previous CDC director, Dr. Robert Redfield, who served during the first year of the pandemic, stated explicitly that "I concur fully with Dr. Kheriaty" that vaccine mandates and passports were unnecessary and unjustified for covid. He stepped down at the CDC shortly before these measures went into effect, and his successor, Dr. Walensky, fully supported vaccine mandates.

For his part Anthony Fauci has acted for over three decades as consummate D.C. politician, styling himself as a scientist and physician, though he has not conducted a scientific experiment or treated a patient for decades. He was praised by George W. Bush and served under several administrations from both parties, craftily using the AIDS epidemic to increase funding for his NIAID division of the NIH. Already in 1989, Fauci organized a conference in D.C. introducing a novel concept of a biosecurity threat.

People had worried about biological weapons prior to 1989, but Fauci's conference introduced a consequential reframing: the potential threat was not a novel *pathogen*, such as a virus or bacteria, whether of natural origin or developed as a bioweapon. Rather, the new paradigm focused instead on *humanity* as a microbial population vector. The challenge was that people functioned as a conveyance apparatus for viruses or bacteria. In other words, the real problem to be addressed was not a virus but a human population that could spread a virus.[83]

The focus shifted accordingly, from finding ways to treat or neutralize a microbial pathogen in those who were sick to finding ways to neutralize the human population that could convey the pathogen. Grasping this point goes a long way towards understanding our failed covid response. On this reconceptualization, humanity, as part of biological nature, must be managed and controlled through strict biomedical security measures. The new solution is not to control or cure a *viral infection* impacting specific people, but to control the *entire population* of human beings. Notice how this reframing subtly pathologizes humanity itself. The human population itself becomes a dangerous problem to be solved by experts—by a new caste of technocrats who must be granted unprecedented powers to control their fellow human beings.

Viral pathogens are not the only imminent threats. The World Economic Forum (WEF), which is working to accelerate the push toward a digital economy, sponsored a cyberattack simulation during covid in July 2020 called Cyber Polygon, the central theme of which was "Digital Pandemic." One of the keynote speakers at this event was former British prime minister Tony Blair, who told participants that a shift to digital identity was inevitable, so governments needed to partner with technology companies on research, development, ands regulation of digital IDs. (We will return to the topic of digital IDs in chapter 3.)

The Cyber Polygon event was repeated with a new script in 2021 and has now become an annual WEF event. A promotional video for the 2021 edition posted on the WEF's YouTube channel warned: "A cyberattack with COVID-like characteristics would spread faster and further than any biological virus. Its reproductive rate would be around 10 times greater than what we've experienced with the coronavirus." The narrator goes on to explain, "As the digital realm increasingly merges with our physical world, the ripple effects of cyber-attacks on our safety just keep on expanding."[84] These annual "digital pandemic" cyber-attack exercises from the WEF, begun in the middle of the covid pandemic, could provide hints about what form our next public health crisis might take.

In every one of these scenarios—as in the real covid pandemic—a coterie of specialized elites moves the levers of the biosecurity apparatus, while the mass of humanity is reconceptualized and dehumanized as a passive population to be managed. In recent years, the term *population health* began replacing the term *public health*, as in UCI's new School of Population Health. Scratching beneath the surface of this subtle change of terminology, we can see that "population" in this context designates a kind of inert mass subjected to external manipulation and control.

Follow the Scientism

History is instructive. Consider the prior regimes in which the pretext of public safety during an emergency paved the way even for totalitarian regimes. Anyone who draws a historical analogy to the Nazis is understandably met with the charge of alarmist hyperbole, so let me be clear: I am comparing neither the current nor the previous administration to Hitler's totalitarian regime. It nevertheless remains a sobering, instructive, and undeniable fact that Nazi Germany was governed for virtually the entirety of its existence under Article 48 of the Weimar Constitution, which allowed for the suspension of German law in times of emergency. The constitutional provision read as follows:

> If public security and order are seriously disturbed or endangered within the German Reich, the President of the Reich may take measures necessary for their restoration, intervening if need be with the assistance of the armed forces. For this purpose he may suspend for a while, in whole or in part, the fundamental rights provided in Articles 114, 115, 117, 118, 123, 124, and 153.[85]

Recall that Hitler was democratically elected. We should ask, How did he manage to go from the elected chancellor to the totalitarian dictator of Germany? A key part of the answer lies in his use of the declared state of emergency. In a similar vein, we should also recall the name of the group that carried out the infamous Reign of Terror during the French Revolution: it was the "Committee on *Public Safety*."

Reaching further back into history we find an instructive lesson from the late Roman Republic. Among the earliest examples of state-sanctioned emergency powers was the provision for the Roman dictator. When the Republic faced an acute existential threat, such as an invading army, the Senate would appoint a dictator with broad powers and the ability to act quickly in a crisis. Even then, there were strict limits: the Senate maintained control of the budget, and dictators faced a strict six-month time limit, with constant pressure to finish the task and retire as soon as the crisis abated. Over a period of three hundred years, dictators were appointed on ninety-five occasions, and each time they were required to quickly relinquish their authority. However, the one time this system failed marked the end of the Roman Republic and the descent into the Empire.[86]

While history does not repeat itself, it often rhymes. This is among the reasons we reach for historical analogies—always imperfect but nevertheless useful—to understand our own time.

If these historical examples seem overblown or unduly alarmist, consider that Australia recently rounded up citizens exposed to covid, including asymptomatic people, and shipped them to detention facilities against their will. Videos of Australian detention centers made their way onto social media before tech censors dutifully scrubbed them from the internet. Many provincial governors in Australia abused their emergency powers: while not every Australian state chose full-throated authoritarianism, several of them did. Canada likewise built detention facilities for infected persons.

Authoritarian measures during the pandemic went beyond detention of suspected or actual cases. The Medical Indemnity Protection Society (MIPS) in Australia provides medical malpractice insurance to all the country's physicians, without which they cannot practice medicine. The MIPS published twelve commandments for physicians on their website to avoid disciplinary "notifications"—an Orwellian euphemism for investigations overseen by the Australian Health Practitioner Regulation

Agency, the governing entity overseeing all physicians. The MIPS commandment number 9 instructed Australian doctors as follows:

> Be very careful when using social media (even on your personal pages), when authoring papers or when appearing in interviews. Health practitioners are obliged to ensure their views are consistent with public health messaging. This is particularly relevant in current times. Views expressed which may be consistent with evidence-based material may not necessarily be consistent with public health messaging.[87]

You might want to read that last sentence one more time. "Evidence-based material" refers to peer-reviewed scientific papers or other sources of credible medical information. So, if Australian doctors mention findings of a published study that are not consistent with "public health messaging"—that is, the views of the public health bureaucrats in power—these physicians could potentially lose their ability to practice medicine. Notice that this applies also to physicians "authoring papers," meaning that if a doctor conducts research and her findings contradict "public health messaging," she'd better think twice before publishing the results. Australia is clearly slouching toward authoritarianism, if not yet totalitarianism.

Likewise, in the United States, the Federation of State Medical Boards (FSMB), an authority on medical licensure and physician discipline, passed a policy in May 2022 on medical misinformation and disinformation that will guide all state medical boards and the nation's physicians they license. This policy may even become state law, as the FSMB recommendations suggest. "More than two years into this pandemic, the largest threat next to the spread of the virus itself is the spread of disinformation and misinformation," FSMB's president and CEO, Humayun Chaudhry, asserted. The policy warns: "Physicians who generate and spread COVID-19 vaccine misinformation or disinformation are risking disciplinary action by state medical boards, including the suspension or revocation of their medical license."

Tellingly, the first example of dangerous misinformation the document cites is physicians not following the FSMB's October 6, 2020, assertion on the efficacy of masks—an assertion later shown to be false: "Wearing a face covering is a harm-reduction strategy to help limit the spread of COVID-19."[88] We will look at the lack of evidence supporting this claim in the final chapter, but for now it's sufficient to note that the question of mask efficacy was still very much in doubt in 2020 when this statement was issued. If the FSMB wanted to address misinformation, they could start with the misinformation their own organization promulgated during the pandemic. They could then move to the falsehoods asserted by our governmental health agencies, who routinely flip-flopped on "The Science." But that's clearly not where the FSMB is aiming its disciplinary rod.

My home state of California took up the FSMB's suggestion to codify these recommendations in law with Assembly Bill 2098. I recently traveled to Sacramento to testify against this legislation in the state senate. The law would empower the state medical board to discipline physicians—including revoking their medical licenses—for spreading misinformation, defined in the law as statements that contradict the current scientific consensus. Undermining its own central claims, the text of AB 2098 made three statements about covid that were already outdated by the time I testified, because science constantly evolves. In my testimony, I argued:

> A physician with a gag order is not a physician you can trust. Advances in science and medicine occur when doctors and scientists challenge conventional thinking or settled opinion. Good science is characterized by conjecture and refutation, lively deliberation, fierce debate, and openness to new data. Thus, fixating any consensus as "unassailable" will stifle medical progress. Frontline physicians challenging conventional thinking played a key role in advancing knowledge of covid treatments. In medicine,

yesterday's minority opinion often becomes today's standard of care. If this bill becomes law, doctors will be punished for practicing medicine according to their best judgment. Informed consent—the foundational principle of ethical medicine—will be compromised.

Following my testimony, the senate committee voted on strict party lines to move the bill to the senate floor, where it is poised to soon be voted into law.

● ● ●

How did we get here? To answer this question, the remainder of this chapter will involve something of a deeper philosophical dive. The Italian philosopher Augusto Del Noce, who came of age in the 1930s and observed with horror the emergence of Mussolini's Fascist regime in his native country, warned that "the widespread notion that the age of totalitarianisms ended with Hitlerism and Stalinism is completely mistaken." He explained:

> The essential element of totalitarianism, in brief, lies in the refusal to recognize the difference between "brute reality" and "human reality," so that it becomes possible to describe man, non-metaphorically, as a "raw material" or as a form of "capital." Today this view, which used to be typical of Communist totalitarianism, has been taken up by its Western alternative, the technological society.[89]

By technological society he did not mean a society characterized by scientific or technological progress, but a society characterized by a view of rationality as purely instrumental. Human reason, on this view, is unable to grasp ideas that go beyond brute empirical facts: we are incapable of discovering transcendent truths. Reason is merely a pragmatic tool, a useful instrument for accomplishing our purposes, but nothing more. Totalitarian ideologies deny that all human beings participate in a shared rationality. We therefore cannot really talk to one another: it is impossible to deliberate or debate civilly in a shared pursuit of truth. Reasoned persuasion has no place. Totalitarian regimes always monopolize what counts as "rational" and therefore what one is permitted to say publicly.

For example, if people in a communist society contradict communist doctrine, the party does not explain why they are wrong. The authorities simply dismiss dissenting opinions as instances of "bourgeois rationality" or "false consciousness." For a communist, if you have not embraced Marx's theory of dialectical materialism, then you do not understand the direction of history. What you are talking about is, by definition, pure nonsense and not worth considering. You are obviously on the "wrong side of history." Authorities assume that dissenting opinions must be motivated by class interests (or racial characteristics, or gender, or whatever), which dissidents are trying to defend.

You don't think such and such because you reasoned logically to that conclusion; you think such and such because you are a white, heterosexual, middle-class American female, and so forth. In this way, totalitarians do not persuade or refute their interlocutors with reasoned arguments. They merely impute bad faith to their opponents and refuse to engage in meaningful debate. They forcibly cut their adversaries off from the sphere of enlightened conversation. One does not bother arguing against such dissidents; one simply steamrolls them after placing them outside the realm of acceptable opinion.

The totalitarianisms of the twentieh century were grounded in pseudoscientific ideologies, for example, the Marxist pseudoscience of economics and history, or the Nazi pseudoscience of race and eugenics. In our own day, the pseudoscientific ideology that drives societies in a totalitarian direction is *scientism*, which must be clearly distinguished from *science*. The ideology of scientism and the practice of science should not be confused: the former is often conflated with the latter, which creates no end of muddled thinking.

Science is a method, or more accurately, a collection of various methods, aimed at systematically investigating observable phenomena in the natural world. Rigorous science is characterized by hypothesis, experiment, testing, interpretation, and ongoing deliberation and debate. Put a group of real scientists in a room together, and they will argue endlessly about the salience, significance, and interpretation of data, about the limitations and strengths of various research methodologies, and about the big picture questions. Science is an enormously complex human enterprise, with each scientific discipline having its own refined methods of inquiry and its own competing theories. Science is not an irrefutable body of knowledge. It is always fallible, always open to revision; yet when conducted rigorously and carefully, scientific research is capable of genuine discoveries and important advances.

Scientism is the philosophical claim—which cannot be proven scientifically—that science is the only valid form of knowledge. Anyone who begins a sentence with the phrase, "Science says . . ." is likely in the grip of scientism. Genuine scientists don't talk like this. They begin sentences with phrases like, "The findings of this study suggest . . ." or, "This meta-analysis concluded . . ." Scientism, by contrast, is a religious and often a political ideology. "It has been evident for quite a while that science has become our time's religion," Agamben observed, "the thing which people believe that they believe in."[90] When science becomes a religion—a closed and exclusionary belief system—we are dealing with scientism.

The characteristic feature of science is warranted uncertainty, which leads to intellectual humility.

The characteristic feature of scientism is unwarranted certainty, which leads to intellectual hubris.

Del Noce realized that *scientism is intrinsically totalitarian*, a profound insight of enormous importance for our time. "Many people do not realize that scientism and the technological society are totalitarian in nature," he wrote fifty years ago.[91] To understand why, consider that scientism and totalitarianism both claim a monopoly on knowledge. The advocate of scientism and the true believer in a totalitarian system both assert that many common-sense notions are simply irrational, unverifiable, unscientific, and therefore outside the scope of what can be said publicly. Antigone's claim, "I have a duty, inscribed indelibly on the human heart, to bury my dead brother," is not a scientific statement; therefore, according to the ideology of scientism, it is pure nonsense.[92] All moral or metaphysical claims are specifically excluded because they cannot be verified by the methods of science or established by the reigning pseudoscientific totalitarian ideology.

Of course, the forced exclusion of moral, metaphysical, or religious claims is not a conclusion of science, but an unprovable philosophical premise of scientism. The assertion that science is the only valid form of knowledge is itself a metaphysical (not a scientific) claim, smuggled in quietly through the backdoor. Scientism needs to hide this self-refuting fact from itself, so it is necessarily mendacious: dishonesty is baked into the system, and various forms of irrationalism follow. The twentieth-century totalitarian ideologies all claimed to be "scientific," but were in fact unfalsifiable by their own circular logic. Because scientism cannot establish itself through rational argument, it relies instead on three tools to advance: brute force, defamation of critics, and the promise of future happiness. These are the same tools deployed by all totalitarian systems.

To hide its own internal contradiction from view, the self-refuting premise of scientism is rarely stated explicitly. Scientism is instead implicitly assumed, its conclusions repeatedly asserted, until this ideology simply becomes the air we breathe. Careful policing of public discourse admits only evidence supposedly supported by "science," and this atmosphere is rigorously enforced. As we will see in the next chapter, during the pandemic, qualitative (for example, familial, spiritual) goods were repeatedly sacrificed to quantitative (for example, biological, medical) goods, even when the former were real and the latter only theoretical.

This is the fruit of scientism, which turns our scale of values and priorities upside down.

It would be hard to find a more effective ideological tool for imposing a totalitarian system than by appealing to "The Science" or "The Experts" and thereby claiming a monopoly on knowledge and rationality. Those in power can readily choose which scientific experts they endorse and which they silence. This allows politicians to defer inescapably political judgments to "The Experts," thus abdicating their own responsibility. One's ideological opponents are hamstrung, their opinions excluded as "unscientific," and their public voice silenced—all without the trouble of maintaining a regime of brute force and physical violence. Defamation and exclusion from public discourse work just as effectively. Those in power maintain a monopoly on what counts as rationality (or science); they do not bother talking to or debating the (fill-in-the-blank stigmatized group) "bourgeois," "Jew," "unvaccinated," "unmasked," "anti-science," or "covid denier," et cetera.

Repressive social conformity is thus achieved without resorting to concentration camps, gulags, the Gestapo, the KGB, or openly despotic tyrants. Instead, dissenters are confined to a moral ghetto through censorship and slander. Recalcitrant individuals are placed outside the purview of polite society and excluded from enlightened conversation. The political theorist Eric Voegelin observed that the essence of totalitarianism is simply that *certain questions are forbidden*.[93] The prohibition against asking questions is a deliberately and skillfully elaborated obstruction of reason in a totalitarian system. If one asks certain questions—Do we really need to continue locking down? or, Are we sure these vaccines are safe and effective? or, Why has the promised utopia not yet arrived?—one will be accused of being a pandemic denier, wanting to kill grandma, being anti-science, or of placing oneself on the "wrong side of history."

We can now appreciate why Del Noce claimed that a technocratic society grounded in scientism is totalitarian, though not obviously authoritarian in the sense of openly violent forms of repression. In a strongly worded passage of an essay titled "The Roots of the Crisis," he made this prediction fifty years ago:

> The remaining believers in a transcendent authority of values will be marginalized and reduced to second-class citizens. They will be imprisoned, ultimately, in "moral" concentration camps. But nobody can seriously think that moral punishments will be less severe than physical punishments. At the end of the process lies the spiritual version of genocide.[94]

In a technocratic society, one ends up in a moral concentration camp if one is not on board with the pseudoscience du jour, the ideological trend of the moment. Whatever questions, concerns, or objections one might raise—whether philosophical, religious, ethical, or simply a different interpretation of scientific evidence—need not be considered. The dissident's questions or opinions do not count; they are ruled out by appeal to "The Science"—trademarked by the regime and printed with a capital *T* and capital *S*.

In another striking passage, written even earlier in 1968, Del Noce warned:

> The de-humanization process that characterized the totalitarian regimes did not stop [after World War II]; it has actually become stronger. "We cannot see its endpoint.". . . Given that every society reflects the people who form it, we are threatened by oligarchies and persecutory systems that would make Nazism and Stalinism look like pale images, although, of course, [these new oligarchies and persecutory systems] will not present themselves as a new Nazism or a new Stalinism.[95]

Given the developments of the last few decades, which manifested with greater clarity during the covid pandemic, we see clearly that the new oligarchies and persecutory systems will present themselves under the banner of *biomedical security measures essential for maintaining population health.* The oligarchs will preface their agenda with phrases like, "Out of an abundance of caution . . ." and "We are all in this together . . ." The new social-distancing societal paradigm facilitates the oligarchs' dominance by separating citizens from one another.

Scientism is a totalitarianism of disintegration before it is a totalitarianism of domination. Recall that lockdowns and social distancing, with their inevitable social isolation, necessarily preceded vaccine mandates and passports, when the repressive regime really tipped its hand. Each of these measures relied on exceptionally sloppy data presented publicly as the only authoritative interpretation of science. In most instances, the pretense of scientific rigor was not even required.

In a scientistic-technocratic regime, the naked individual—reduced to "bare biological life," cut off from other people and from anything transcendent—becomes completely dependent on society. The human person, reduced to a free-floating, untethered, and uprooted social atom, is more readily manipulated. Del Noce made the startling claim that scientism is even more opposed to tradition than communism, because in Marxist ideology we still find messianic and biblical archetypes dimly represented in the promise of a future utopia.[96] By contrast, "scientistic anti-traditionalism can express itself only by dissolving the 'fatherlands' where it was born." This process leaves the entire field of human life wide open to domination by global corporations and their suborned political agents:

> Because of the very nature of science, which provides means but does not determine any ends, scientism lends itself to be used as a tool by some group. Which group? The answer is completely obvious: once the fatherlands are gone, all that is left are the great economic organisms, which look more and more like fiefdoms. States become their executive instruments.[97]

States as instruments of world-spanning corporations, which operate like fiefdoms, is an apt definition of corporatism, as we will see in chapter 3. In this global non-society, individuals are radically uprooted and instrumentalized. The ultimate result, in the last analysis, is pure nihilism: "After the negation of every possible authority of values, all that is left is pure total negativism, and the will for something so indeterminate that it is close to 'nothing,'" in Del Noce's bleak description.[98] This is clearly a society suited neither to a meaningful human life nor to social harmony.

● ● ●

The technocratic society, with scientism as its public theology, is not the inevitable consequence of scientific advance or technological progress. This bears repeating: progress in science and advances in technology are not the source of our crisis. The problem is the mischaracterization of science as the only valid authority, the enthronement of science as the exclusive reigning principle for all knowledge and for all of society. This ideology rests upon a particular interpretation of contemporary history implicit in scientism's founding myth. It is not the pursuit of science or technology as such, but a myth of progress via radical rupture with the past, that lies at the root of our technocratic society and its totalitarian threat.

Del Noce described this myth as follows: "What motivates the criticism of tradition and all its consequences is the millennialist idea of a sharp break in history leading to a radically new type of civilization."[99] Scientism is founded on a revolutionary utopian dream that destroys everything that came before in preparation for a totally different future. This interpretation of contemporary history began to take hold in Western countries in the decades following the Second World War; but the idea accelerated dramatically during the pandemic.

Overcoming scientism requires recovering an accurate and balanced sense of contemporary history. This includes an awareness that the horrors of the last century were born not from tradition but precisely from the myth of total novelty—the myth of a complete revolutionary rupture with the past—the same myth that characterized all the totalitarianisms of the twentieth century. Marxism, fascism, Nazism, and even the eugenics movement all adopted their own versions of this story of total revolutionary rupture. Scientism—and its misbegotten child, transhumanism, which we will encounter later—likewise presents its own version of a radical rupture from the past.

It's worth briefly describing how this myth functioned in totalitarian ideologies of the past hundred years, so that we can better appreciate how it functions in today's totalitarian threat. It is easy to see in Marxist thought the idea of a sharp rupture with previous history: the doctrine of the communist revolution posits a radical break from the past, which will usher us into a realm so entirely new that it is difficult to describe in words. Little more needs to be said about the communist example. At first glance, however, this myth of radical rupture may not be so clear in fascism and Nazism.

Regarding fascism, in his will to dominate, Mussolini spontaneously identified himself with the fatherland and with his own people. At first glance, this sounds vaguely like an embrace of "tradition" or a nostalgia for the national past. However, there was no trace in Mussolini's Fascist doctrine of any actual tradition that he admired or defended. Contrary to popular mischaracterizations, fascism made no attempt to preserve a heritage of traditional values against the advance of progress. One only needs to look at the disruptive "futuristic" novelty in Italian Fascist architecture for confirmation of this. Fascist ideology always presented itself as the unfolding in history of a wholly novel and unprecedented power.

Fascism was therefore not a reactionary-traditionalist movement, but a rival cousin of Marxist revolutionary thought. As Ernst Nolte has documented, there was both a "mysterious proximity and distance between Mussolini and Lenin."[100] In the 1920s Mussolini was constantly glancing over his shoulder at Lenin as a rival disruptive revolutionary in a kind of mimetic dance. Both fascism and communism grew from the same revolutionary root: each proposed a radical rupture from the past as its necessary precondition. Rather than looking back to history or to transhistorical values, fascism strained forward and advanced by means of "creative destruction": it felt entitled to overturn everything standing in its way.

Action for its own sake took on a particular aura and mystique, just as disruptive forms of innovation do today in Silicon Valley. The fascist ideologue, like the technocratic ideologue today, unflinchingly appropriates various sources of energy—human, cultural, religious, or technical—to remake and transform reality. As fascism advances it makes no attempt to conform to any higher truth or transcendent moral order. Mirroring what we will see in the third chapter when we examine the transhumanists, for the fascist, reality is simply that which must be overcome. For both fascism and transhumanism, nature is nothing more than inert raw material to be reshaped by technology.

What about Nazism? The Nazi party developed its own origin story, but this story was not tied to any actual European history: Nazism's Aryan racial doctrine necessarily had to ground itself in a mythic *prehistory*. As with fascism and communism, Nazism was always ahistorical and entirely uninterested in preserving anything meaningful from the past.[101] Nazism was simply the Marxist revolution in reverse: instead of a communist dream of *universal* socialism, Nazi doctrine proposed a blood-and-soil *National* Socialism. Whatever their differences, both ideologies clearly led to extreme forms of colonialism and aggressive destruction in their efforts to create a radically new society.

In summary, all three of these totalitarian ideologies—communism, fascism, and Nazism—were rotten fruits from the same bad tree. Though they differed in important respects, all three were grounded in a myth of radical revolutionary rupture with the past; all three promised an entirely new future; all three entailed the wholesale rejection of any transcendent source of moral authority. We find these same features in the ideology of scientism.

A genuine historical awareness allows us to question the idols of our scientistic-technocratic society. This society has become focused exclusively on purely material wellbeing, understood as the increase of vitality and the preservation of bare biological life. There is nothing "scientific" about enshrining raw vitality and bare life as our highest goods, at the expense of all other human and spiritual goods. There is nothing "scientific" about ignoring such universal human goods as family, friendship, community, knowledge, beauty, worship, devotion, virtue, God, and so on.

● ● ●

Mattias Desmet—whose theory of mass formation was recently popularized by my colleague Dr. Robert Malone on Joe Rogan's podcast—points out that there are key differences between a dictatorship and a totalitarian society.[102] In a dictatorship people obey the ruling authority because they are afraid of the power of the dictator. By contrast totalitarianism begins with the process of mass formation, which creates an emotionally strong social bond. In the hypnotic atmosphere of the mass, most citizens tend to internalize the power and rules of the state in ways not seen in a classical dictatorship. Dictators rule from without while totalitarians rule from within.[103]

The enslavement of populations in a totalitarian regime is stronger and harder to break because those who have internalized the totalitarian constraints do not realize they are enslaved. Already during the pandemic, we transformed from relatively free and responsible citizens in a participatory democracy to a crowd, a mass, a collection of raw material praised only for our plasticity. Unlike a dense mass pressed together at a rock concert, social distancing rules made us into a non-dense, rarified mass—a mass whose elements kept themselves apart at all costs—but still a mass, nevertheless, as defined by our passivity, uniformity, and pliability.

In a passage that ties together several of our themes, the philosopher Giorgio Agamben summarizes the essential elements of the biomedical security apparatus now in place—elements that produce entirely new forms of governance and social life that he dubs the Great Transformation:

> If the juridical-political apparatus of the Great Transformation is the *state of exception*, and the religious apparatus is science [science as religion = *scientism*], on the social plane this transformation relied for its efficacy upon *digital technology* which, as is now evident, works in harmony with the new structure of relationships known as *"social distancing."* Human relationships will have to happen, on every occasion and as much as possible, without physical presence. They will be relegated—much as was already happening—to digital devices that are becoming increasingly efficacious and pervasive. The new model of social relations is [purely digital] connection, and whoever is not connected tends to be excluded from relationships and condemned to marginalisation [emphasis added].[104]

The interlocking of these mechanisms—the state of emergency and its associated police powers, a militarized public health apparatus, science presented as a religious ideology, and surveillance and information control via digital technologies—has already produced a modern Leviathan. We are only beginning to feel the effects of its power.

If the rising biomedical security state does not meet robust resistance in the years ahead, we can be sure it will force increasingly onerous burdens on our lives and intrusive interventions into our bodies. In this paradigm for a wholly transformed society, ruptured from the past and uprooted from the present, citizens are no longer viewed as persons with inherent dignity. Instead, we are merely fungible elements of an undifferentiated mass, to be shaped by supposedly benevolent health-and-safety "experts" who know nothing outside of state-sanctioned opinion.

The unholy alliance of a militarized, global public health regime and its state of exception with digital technologies of surveillance, personal-data extraction, information flow, and social control makes possible extraordinarily granular forms of domination unimaginable by the totalitarian regimes of the past. Whether we agree or disagree with this or that public policy (for example, a vaccine mandate), this broader issue of surveillance and control should concern everyone. The biomedical security state will leave no aspect of our individual and common life untouched.

Perhaps even more tragic than the loss of freedoms in the recent transformation was the decay and deterioration of genuine human relationships, which dissolve in the crowd or mass. Agamben asks whether such a society can still define itself as human, "or if the loss of sensible relationships, of the face, of friendship, of love, can truly be compensated for by an abstract and presumably absolutely fictitious health security."[105] As we have experienced during the pandemic, families were often torn asunder and friendships were frequently sacrificed under the enormous pressure of our destructive pandemic policies and our collective fear.

These are the early fruits of The New Abnormal. If we do not soon change course, there is much more to come. Why am I convinced of this? In 2021 I found myself ground through the gears of the biomedical security apparatus. My experiences trying to resist this machinery changed my entire career as an academic physician and medical ethicist. My personal story, which I tell in the next chapter, illustrates how the biomedical security state took visible form during the covid pandemic.

CHAPTER 2

Locked Down & Locked Out: A New Societal Paradigm

The whole earth is our hospital
Endowed by the ruined millionaire,
Wherein, if we do well, we shall
Die of the absolute paternal care
That will not leave us, but prevents us everywhere.

—*T. S. Eliot, "East Coker"*

In 2021 we conducted the largest experiment on human subjects in world history. Without informed consent. That experiment failed.

In the waning weeks of that year, I found myself in the national-media spotlight. The headline "University ethics professor fired for challenging the ethics of the University's vaccine mandate" grabbed the attention of a weary and worried public, bruised and bullied by authoritarian and illogical pandemic policies. In January 2022 I stood on the steps of the Lincoln Memorial to address a crowd of forty thousand people. We had gathered in the nation's capital in frigid twenty-degree weather to oppose overbearing covid restrictions and coercive policies. Glancing down, I noticed a marble slab adjacent to the podium commemorating Martin Luther King Jr.'s "I Have a Dream" speech, delivered on that exact spot fifty years ago. The next day I testified on a panel at the U.S. Senate to provide a "second opinion" on our covid pandemic response. In this chapter, I will recount the backstory of how I got there, as well as my legal battles with the CDC and the FDA.

In my remarks at the Lincoln Memorial, I reminded those gathered for the first "Defeat the Mandates" march that the issues we faced were about much more than lockdowns or vaccine mandates and passports. These were merely early steps in the advance of a wholly new paradigm that would impact all of society: "We are seeing the emergence of a new biosecurity surveillance regime run by unelected technocrats," I explained. "The welding of digital technologies, public health, and police power is leading to unprecedented invasions on our privacy and intrusive methods of monitoring and authoritarian control." We will see how the initial stages of this infrastructure were implemented during the pandemic.

"Your Papers, Please"

In 2021 covid vaccine mandates were harnessed to a novel system of vaccine passports and digital surveillance that turned many jurisdictions into discriminatory "papers, please" regimes. The omicron wave late in the year demonstrated the failure of mandates and passports to slow the spread of the virus. By March 2022 these measures were abandoned in many places, but mandates remained at some institutions like the University of California, where I worked. Although most jurisdictions eased off vaccine passports, the proof-of-concept experiment had already been demonstrated.

Let's examine how vaccine passports functioned. In December 2021 a relative of mine, who will remain unnamed, went to a Sacramento Kings basketball game. There were three lines to get into the arena: (1) proof of vaccination, (2) rapid covid test, and (3) proof of recent negative test. He was vaccinated and could show his digital vaccine passport to prove this, but he figured he'd get a rapid test just to see if he had covid. He tested positive. So he promptly walked from the rapid test line into the vaccinated line, showed his vaccine passport, and went into the game.

Two months prior, in September 2021, three black women went to eat at Carmine's, an upscale restaurant in Manhattan. The hostess asked to see the vaccine passports of the men accompanying them, vaccine passports the men did not have. An altercation ensued between the women and the hostess. The police were called to the scene. Despite physically aggressive actions caught on camera from both the black women and the white host, only the women of color were arrested. The *New York Times* reported that the hostess allegedly used a racial slur and spoke condescendingly to the patrons, suggesting that their vaccine cards were fake.[1]

Throughout the mass vaccination campaign, we knew that blacks—having historically understandable reasons for mistrusting our public health establishment—remained disproportionately unvaccinated. This made vaccine passports, like the eugenics policies described in the prologue, a de facto form of racial discrimination. The three women simply trying to eat at a decent Manhattan restaurant were punished for resisting the insidiously designed racial and class-based segregation policy of vaccine passports.

Societal exclusion was baked into the system. Policymakers openly admitted that the intent of vaccine passports was to make life so uncomfortable for the unvaccinated that they would eventually fall in line and get the jab. In entirely foreseeable ways, these policies entrenched discriminatory practices under the thin veneer of public health. Worries among blacks about the discriminatory effects of these policies were not assuaged by New York's approach to mass vaccination. As the *New York Times* reported in August 2021:

> One of the three vaccines—the single-shot Johnson & Johnson—had been directed to Black and Latino communities, among other places. It required only one shot—not two like the Moderna and Pfizer vaccines—and had less onerous refrigeration requirements. It struck many government officials as the obvious choice for the pop-up vaccine clinics at public

housing projects and churches that were central to the government's plan for vaccinating minority neighborhoods.[2]

This vaccine was less efficacious than the other two according to the clinical trials data submitted to the FDA. In February 2021 the federal government temporarily halted its use over reports of blood clots, and the following year the FDA recommended that, due to ongoing concerns about thrombosis, the J&J shot should only be used for people who could not take the other vaccines. By then, however, it had already been widely deployed as the vaccine of choice for minority populations. These revelations did not, as you can imagine, restore blacks' trust in the public health establishment.

But the disparate impacts of vaccine passports were only one of their many serious defects. For more than a year, ordinary people accepted, as a routine condition of traveling, working, and accessing public spaces, a system of surveillance and control that would have been unthinkable only a few years ago. Before the pandemic, if anyone had seriously proposed setting up checkpoints where citizens had to show a QR code demonstrating that they had accepted the injection of a novel vaccine—with the attendant release of private health information to a stranger—to get on a plane, board a train, go to a restaurant, attend a public gathering, or get back into their own country, citizens would have immediately revolted. The deployment of fear during covid created a social and psychological climate in which citizens conceded to this system of surveillance and control with little resistance.

Freedom of movement, of association, of domicile in one's country of origin, and access to public spaces and public events—these quickly went from basic rights to special privileges conferred by governments as rewards for good behavior. The transformation of these rights into privileges required the enormous strain of prolonged lockdowns followed by the promise of vaccination as the only ticket back to a normal life. People accepted this bargain under conditions of psychological duress. After the repetitive trauma of rolling lockdowns, most citizens were willing to do just about anything if it meant a return to those aspects of normal social life that had been suddenly stripped away.

Most countries in Europe, as well as many cities and counties in the United States, implemented vaccine passport systems in 2021. Australia, Canada, New Zealand, Japan, Uruguay, and Argentina likewise embraced vaccine passports. These were not only required to travel, access public buildings, and qualify for basic services, but even to work within one's own country of residence.[3] This system exacerbated the two-tiered society that lockdowns helped create, worsening social divisions and stigmatizing large segments of the population.

Vaccine passport systems were not invented on the spot to deal with covid: plans for these preceded the pandemic. For example, the European Union's Green Pass vaccine certificate was gestated in 2018, more than a year before the first covid case. The EU's plan was for a vaccine passport for all citizens by 2022, but the pandemic accelerated this process, and these objectives were already met by 2021. During covid, without the EU's Green Pass—implemented on June 1, 2021, by twenty-seven member states—Italians could not work, and in many other European countries citizens could not access public services or education. The Green Pass was necessary to go to restaurants, bars, museums, supermarkets, gyms, libraries, and other public places. The EU's vaccine passport functioned as a system of incredibly harsh exclusion.[4]

The definition of "fully vaccinated" became a moving target with the rollout of boosters, such that access granted by a vaccine passport was given only temporarily. Ironically, this was exacerbated by the failure of vaccines to provide long-term protection against the virus and by the unfounded hope that additional doses would remedy these deficiencies, though there was little to no data to support this. Booster mandates were a reminder that these passports were not in fact *passports*, which have a predetermined expiration date that does not change. Vaccine "passports" were actually temporary licenses for living: the government's permission to move and participate in civil society could be rescinded at any moment.

A passport is a document that allows one to enter a foreign country. We don't need permission to leave our own country: one can go up in a plane or balloon, or sail the ocean blue, as far from home as one wants. If you build a rocket ship, you can go to the moon. One needs permission, however, to land on foreign soil. Thus, if vaccine passports really are passports, they turn every person into an alien in his or her own homeland. This represents, quite literally, the most alienating domestic policy ever devised. Under a vaccine passport regime, we are all homeless, every one of us an exile, a stranger in a strange land. To deny that vaccine passports do this is to admit that they are not passports but are instead, as I suggested, temporary licenses to live.

A vaccine passport was never a reliable indicator of immune status, transmission risk to others, or any other relevant covid metric. If the lack of a vaccine passport indicated anything at all, it was a tendency toward nonconformity. These licenses to live are a vivid example of what French philosopher Michel Foucault called "the penetration of regulation into even the smallest details of everyday life."[5] There was never any evidence when these were implemented, and there remains no evidence today that the vaccine passport regime improved public health outcomes. That citizens never demanded any evidence before acceding to this regime is a worrisome sign of the times.

Indeed, there is plenty of evidence that vaccine passports failed to mitigate viral spread. The Boardmasters Music Festival in the United Kingdom in August 2021 resulted in an outbreak of five thousand covid cases the following week, amounting to 10 percent of all attendees, despite requiring the NHS vaccine pass to attend. Harvard Business School likewise did everything by the book and nevertheless had an outbreak of sixty cases within a few weeks of the beginning of their 2021 fall semester, even though 95 percent of students and 96 percent of faculty were vaccinated. In July 2021 the British HMS *Queen Elizabeth* had an outbreak of one hundred cases despite a 100 percent vaccination rate among the passengers and crew.[6] A 2021 study from Harvard researchers, which received no attention in the media, found that "increases in COVID-19 are unrelated to vaccination levels across 68 countries and 2947 counties in the United States."[7]

Vaccine efficacy had been clearly declining for months by summer 2021; by the time the omicron wave hit late in the year, vaccines were useless against infection. One study on vaccine immunity for omicron showed zero vaccine efficacy for the full two-dose regimen of the mRNA vaccines (Pfizer or Moderna) against this variant. After giving a third booster dose, the study found that vaccine efficacy against omicron was 37 percent, far below the 50 percent efficacy threshold set by the FDA for vaccine approval. This peak efficacy declined by eight weeks, even faster than efficacy from the initial two-dose regimen declined.[8] Consistent with these findings, the World Health Organization (WHO) announced in September 2021 that a strategy of repeated boosters was likely not feasible and would introduce ongoing repeated risks of vaccine adverse effects.[9]

Even worse, by early 2022 many highly vaccinated and boosted regions around the world—including, for example, Israel, Ontario Canada, England, and Scotland—showed data suggesting negative vaccine efficacy.[10] For example, a study from Qatar published in the in the *New England Journal of Medicine* in June 2022 showed negative vaccine efficacy against omicron infection.[11] This meant not just a failure of vaccines to offer protection against infection or transmission, but an *increased* rate of infection among the vaccinated compared to the unvaccinated.

Data from states like Vermont showed a similar trend. However, we could not be entirely certain exactly where negative efficacy was occurring in the United States because, as the *New York Times* reported in February 2022, the CDC was withholding or delaying the public release of much of its data on cases, hospitalizations, and deaths. The stated reason from the CDC spokesperson gave the game away: the agency was concerned that their data might increase "vaccine hesitancy." As the article reported, "The C.D.C. has been routinely collecting information since the Covid vaccines were first rolled out last year, according to a federal official familiar with the effort. The agency has been reluctant to make those figures public, the official said, because they might be misinterpreted as the vaccines being ineffective."[12] Instead of altering vaccine policies when new data contradicted them, public health agencies buried the data to save the policies.

Meanwhile, Britain was still releasing its data, and it did not look good. By March 2022 nearly 95 percent of all adults were fully vaccinated, including close to 100 percent of seniors, with 90 percent of seniors boosted. Yet for individuals over the age of seventy, infections hit record highs. Scotland, which had the highest vaccination rate of anywhere in the United Kingdom and was the only region with mask mandates, was doing worse than ever: "Scotland recorded its highest infection rates of the pandemic so far, with one in every 14 people infected with the virus in the week to mid-March, up from one in 18 a week earlier," the *Financial Times* reported. The boosted accounted for 90 percent of cases among the elderly, whereas just 1.6 percent of cases among the elderly were in the unvaccinated, though they accounted for 5 percent of that cohort. Fifteen percent of all the deaths were among the double-jabbed, though they accounted for only 4 percent of the population.[13]

The death counts looked so bad that Scotland also stopped providing that data, concerned that it would increase vaccine hesitancy.[14] As in the United States, they buried data to save the policies. The United Kingdom was seeing evidence of what other highly vaccinated regions like Israel and Ontario had seen a month or two earlier. The vaccines were not just failing to prevent infections, data suggested they were increasing the odds of infection. There were at least two possible explanations for this. Thoughtful scientists had raised these as potential problems with these vaccines from the beginning. Their concerns were ignored, even though both issues had bedeviled vaccine production for other viruses like HIV.

The first explanation was antigenic imprinting, also known as "original antigenic sin." In this process, the vaccine focuses the immune system's response too narrowly on only one antigen (or part of the virus), in this case the original spike protein from the Wuhan strain, which by 2022 was no longer in circulation. This could suppress the broad-based natural immunity, with balanced responses from the humoral (B cell) and cellular (T cell) branches of the immune system, which would be generally effective against new variants. Rather than shooting a bird in flight with a shotgun that sprays broadly (our immune system's innate immunity or natural immunity following infection), the vaccines trained the system to fire from a single-shot rifle that easily misses the moving target.

The second explanation for negative vaccine efficacy was antibody dependent enhancement. This involves binding of suboptimal antibodies, in this case the antibodies to the original spike protein, that are a poor fit for new variants of this protein. This paradoxically enhances entry of the virus into human cells, facilitating infection and viral replication. We had already seen this happen with the swine flu (H_1N_1) vaccine and with the Dengue virus, among other pathogens. The spike protein was evolving precisely to evade vaccine immunity, and several eminent virologists warned that this problem was likely to occur. The public health establishment ignored these warnings.

These two possibilities were not mutually exclusive: both could form part of the explanation for the trends of early 2022. Even if it was unclear *why* we were seeing this problem emerge, *that* we were seeing it was increasingly undeniable, though plenty of people still tried to ignore it. By early 2022 it was well past time to rethink the mass vaccination campaign. With each passing month, the failure of these coercive vaccine mandates and passports to achieve their aims—and the harms they inflicted—became more apparent.

While courts in the United States struck down some vaccine mandates, and many jurisdictions around the world abandoned them voluntarily, other leaders—from Justin Trudeau to Governor Newsom to the president of the University of California (UC)—refused to pivot in the face of accumulating evidence. Instead, they doubled down on failed policies. The UC vaccine mandate, like so many others, became a booster mandate in January 2022. Faculty, staff, and students who thought they would be left alone if they gave in to the first mandate were in for a rude awakening. By April 2022 students at UCI, where I had spent my entire career, had their Wi-Fi turned off if they still were not boosted, and the university was threatening expulsion.[15] Many faculty and students reached out to me at that time and expressed that, while they reluctantly took the initial doses so they could remain at the university, they would draw the line at forced boosters.

*   *   *

In their understandable enthusiasm to rollout the novel covid vaccines as widely and quickly as possible in early 2021, the public health establishment succumbed to two dangerous temptations: propaganda and coercion. That their approach deployed these with the common good in mind (achieving herd immunity) and with good intentions (ending the pandemic as quickly as possible) does not alter the fact that such approaches were deeply misguided and represented deeply disturbing trends in public policy. These trends stemmed from the same scientistic ideology undergirding the biomedical security model: public pronouncements in the name of science could not be questioned, and behavioral outcomes could be achieved by any means necessary.

Coercive covid vaccination mandates rested on several unproven postulates, which mainstream opinion took to be axiomatic and unassailable: (1) the vaccines are safe for everyone; (2) the vaccines are necessary for everyone; therefore, (3) any vaccine hesitancy is a public relations problem that must be overcome. The "needle in every arm" goal was set in advance; the only deliberation permitted was about the most efficient means toward this predetermined end. Any scientist, physician, or policymaker who broke ranks to question one or more of these axioms was at best a nuisance or at worst dangerous—someone to be ignored as backwards or dismissed as a threat to public health. People who asked inconvenient questions were labeled with the dismissive "anti-vax" epithet, a term that functioned to exclude them from the realm of reasonable discourse.

After moving the goalposts several times on the percentage of the population that needed to be vaccinated to achieve herd immunity, Anthony Fauci's subsequent remarks about vaccination in 2021 became masterworks of misdirection: "We should not get so fixated on this elusive number of herd immunity," Fauci said in March that year. "We should just be concerned about getting as many people vaccinated as quickly as we possibly can because herd immunity is still somewhat of an elusive number."[16] Again, in April that year he referred to herd immunity as a "mystical elusive number."[17] He could perhaps forgive the mysticism of Americans who embraced the notion of herd immunity. After all for an entire year public health officials had repeatedly drummed into our heads the idea that herd immunity was our golden ticket out of lockdowns.

Some of the vaccine propaganda would have been laughable if it wasn't so clearly displaying sanctimonious contempt for its audience. Consider a televised public service announcement from Ohio's Department of Health: a friendly immunologist clears up misinformation about what's in a covid vaccine by explaining, "There's just a few simple ingredients: water, sugar, salt, fat, and most importantly, a building block for protein. . . . That's less stuff than a candy bar or a can of pop."[18] The absurd message suggests that vaccine risks are no different from the risks of eating a candy bar or drinking a soda—clearly government-sponsored misinformation if that word means anything. The condescension on display also tells you all you need to know about what Ohio's public health officials think of the intelligence of the average citizen.

Aside from what was said, the most egregious form of propaganda was the vaccine-related information that was deliberately withheld or deemphasized. As mentioned earlier, the *New York Times* reported in March 2022: "Two full years into the pandemic, the agency leading the country's response to the public health emergency [the CDC] has published only a tiny fraction of the data it has collected." For example, when the agency "published the first significant data on the effectiveness of boosters in adults younger than 65 . . . it left out the numbers for a huge portion of that population: 18- to 49-year-olds, the group least likely to benefit from extra shots." The CDC's stated reason for withholding much of its data was that it did not want to increase vaccine hesitancy.[19]

The result was messaging from public health officials that sounded indistinguishable from the marketing departments of Pfizer, Moderna, and Johnson & Johnson. Granted, public health communications must be simplified for broad consumption; but there is a key difference between simplifying information for the layperson and dumbing it down to manipulate the masses or deliberately suppressing information that might undermine a predetermined public policy. This was not public education but a manipulative effort at behavioral control. In the most precise meaning of the term, it was propaganda. Large swaths of the public who were not hypnotized by the repetition of memes could sense, even if they could not explain, that they were subjected to manipulation.

As vaccination rates approached 50 percent in the United States, vaccine uptake slowed by April 2021. Reports began to emerge of serious side effects, and studies from Israel, which started its mass vaccination campaign before the United States, suggested that vaccine efficacy waned rapidly. Public health efforts pivoted from propaganda to heavy-handed nudges and bribes. Several states entered vaccinated citizens into lotteries awarding cash prizes of $1 million or more. Other states and cities launched promotions for vaccination ranging from free beer in New Jersey to raffles for full-ride college scholarships in New York and Ohio to a free marijuana joint in Washington for those who took the jab.[20] (The latter brought to you, naturally, by people who sincerely care about your health.)

When these nudges didn't work, officials simply mandated the vaccines, with severe penalties for those who declined. As my own institution, the University of California, prepared to issue its vaccine mandate, I argued publicly in the pages of the *Wall Street Journal* in June 2021 that university vaccine mandates violated foundational principles of medical ethics, including the principle of informed consent described in the prologue. Although the minimal conditions for justifying vaccine mandates were never close to being met, institutions embraced these misguided policies with little meaningful public discussion and no debate. I wrote at the time: "We must maintain our integrity under pressure. It is precisely in dire situations, such as wars or pandemics, that we are most sorely tempted to abandon ethical principles. Authorities rushing to implement mandatory vaccination protocols are ignoring available scientific data, basic principles of immunology and elementary [ethical] norms."[21]

Along with my coauthor, professor of law Gerry Bradley, I pointed out that even soldiers, whose rights are constrained when they join the military, were not being compelled to take a covid vaccine when universities embarked on this reckless policy. "In a case involving a vaccine against anthrax, a federal district judge held in 2004 that 'the United States cannot demand that members of the armed forces also serve as guinea pigs for experimental drugs,' absent informed consent or a presidential waiver of service members' legal protections. The following year the judge held that an emergency-use authorization from the FDA was insufficient to meet the legal test."[22]

However, immediately following the FDA authorization of the Pfizer vaccine—though the authorized product Comirnaty was still unavailable in the United States—the military likewise mandated vaccines for its service members. Months later, physician whistleblowers at the Department of Defense (DoD) revealed that the military database we use to monitor health of our troops showed massive harms to our military population coinciding with the rollout of the novel vaccines. We forcibly administered these products to young, healthy members of the armed forces who were not at significant risk from covid.

According to evidence presented at a U.S. Senate panel by attorney Tom Renz, who represented the whistleblowers, the DoD database showed unprecedented spikes in adverse events, including death, during the vaccine mandate period in 2021.[23] This was consistent with the many early safety signals seen in the Vaccine Adverse Events Reporting System (VAERS) and consistent with spikes in all-cause mortality among working-age adults that were later revealed by life-insurance actuarial data. Those red flags still warrant additional follow-up studies, but the only safety issue that received attention from the CDC was myocarditis.

At this same Senate panel, where I also testified, I described the censorious climate surrounding vaccine mandates: "The scientific method suffered from a repressive academic and social climate of censorship and silencing of competing perspectives. This projected the false appearance of a scientific consensus—a 'consensus' often strongly influenced by economic and political interests." I pointed out that vaccine mandates ignored the huge number of people who had already recovered from covid infection and who therefore had infection-induced natural immunity, which studies showed was more robust and durable than vaccine immunity. While vaccinating covid-recovered patients might produce an antibody uptick, there was no epidemiological evidence that this "hybrid immunity" improved relevant clinical outcomes like reinfection or transmissibility.[24]

In the climate of severe censorship, among the few public figures trying to explain these basic scientific facts in 2021 were, to my surprise, several NBA players. The most articulate among them was Jonathan Isaac, the young star forward for the Orlando Magic. In a press conference, Isaac displayed remarkable composure and poise under pressure, describing what we knew about natural immunity, as well as vaccine safety and efficacy, better than most so-called public health experts and other talking heads on television. Impressed with both his courage and intelligence, I reached out to Jonathan, and we struck up a collaborative friendship.

After the *New York Times* mentioned both of us in an article about vaccinating those with natural immunity, Jonathan and I responded by publishing a coauthored piece, "COVID Mandates Prevent Americans from Getting Back in the Game." We clarified the science of hybrid immunity and argued that we could fight covid and defend our liberties simultaneously. As we observed, "The scientific evidence does not favor vaccination—nor warrant coercive mandates or restrictions—for those with natural (infection-induced) immunity. Furthermore, we affirm that all people should maintain the right to informed consent or refusal for COVID vaccines." We also explained:

> The argument that "you might not benefit but should still get vaccinated for the sake of others" does not apply to COVID vaccines, because they do not prevent infection and transmission, but only lower the risk of severe symptoms. There are now countless documented cases of breakthrough infections in the vaccinated, and their likelihood of transmitting the virus is the same as the unvaccinated, as the Director of the CDC has acknowledged. By contrast, there is not a single reported case of someone with natural immunity getting a reinfection and transmitting the virus to others: we are the safest people to be around.

In the closing paragraph, we noted, "The same essential people who courageously worked on the frontlines defending us during COVID now face bullying from their peers and no support from the government of a country that was founded on freedom."[25] By the time I published this piece, I had already personally experienced the illogic and injustice of covid vaccine mandates, as I will recount later in this chapter.

Ground Zero

From the lepers in the Old Testament to the Plague of Justinian in ancient Rome to the 1918 Spanish flu pandemic, covid represents the first time in the history of pandemics that we confined healthy populations. While the ancients did not understand the mechanisms of infectious disease—they knew nothing of viruses and bacteria—they nevertheless figured out many ways to mitigate the spread of contagion during epidemics. These time-tested measures ranged from quarantining symptomatic patients to enlisting those with natural immunity, who had recovered from the illness, to care for the sick.[26]

Lockdowns were never part of conventional public health measures. The concept of lockdowns arose in part from a public health apparatus that had become militarized over the previous two decades. We now routinely hear of "pandemic countermeasures"; but doctors and nurses never speak of viral "countermeasures," which is a term of spy craft and soldiering. In 1968, while an estimated one to four million people died in the H2N3 influenza pandemic, businesses and schools stayed open and large events were never canceled. Until 2020 we had not locked down entire populations, because this strategy does not work. In 2020 we had zero empirical evidence that lockdowns would save lives, only flawed mathematical models whose predications were not just slightly off, but wildly exaggerated by orders of magnitude.

When Drs. Fauci and Birx, leading the president's coronavirus task force, decided in February 2020 that lockdowns were the way to go, the *New York Times* was tasked with explaining this approach to Americans. On February 27 the *Times* published a podcast that opened with science reporter Donald McNeil explaining that the virus appeared to have an infection fatality rate of 2.5 percent. His advice for a worst-case scenario ran as follows: "Mentally prepare yourself for what would happen if you and all of your friends had to stay home for a month, or not be able to ride the subways, or supermarkets ran low on food. Or, you know, your medicine—your insulin or your H.I.V. meds or your heart meds or whatever it is you take—wasn't available because the supply lines from China have been cut off." He also warned that we may run out of ventilators for those who would need them. McNeil then explained the possibility of lockdowns, following China's strategy: "What happened in China, with the shutdown of Wuhan and Hubei province . . . was the equivalent of shutting down Chicago and most of that surrounding part of the Midwest at Christmas time and telling people, you are now going to stay in Chicago. You can't leave. You can't see your families. All the flights are canceled. All the trains are canceled. All the highways are closed. You're going to stay in there. And you're locked in with a deadly disease. We can do it."

The following day, the *Times* published McNeil's article, "To Take On the Coronavirus, Go Medieval on It."[27] The article did not give enough credit to medieval society, which sometimes locked the gates of walled cities or closed borders during epidemics, but never ordered people to stay in their homes, never stopped people from plying their trade, and never isolated asymptomatic individuals from others in the community. No, Mr. McNeil, lockdowns were not a medieval throwback but a wholly modern invention. In March of 2020, lockdowns were an entirely de novo experiment, untested on human populations.

Although these measures were unprecedented, there was virtually no public conversation or debate about lockdown policies. Wise solutions to vexing policy questions always involve prudential judgments that no single epidemiological model can provide. In the first months of the pandemic, we needed leaders willing to navigate those hard judgments. Instead, our politicians abdicated responsibility by hiding behind "The Science" or "The Experts," as though these trademarked phrases conjured a single monolithic table of all-encompassing data. Our leaders should have considered the various complex risks and harms—not to mention a thousand other imponderables—of decisions like lockdowns or mask mandates. With a few notable exceptions, most of our leadership class failed spectacularly. Even now, they remain unwilling to admit their mistakes.

It's hard to overstate the novelty and folly of what happened worldwide in March 2020. We were introduced not just to a new and previously untested method of infection control. More than this, we embraced a new paradigm for society—one that had been decades in the making, but that would have been impossible just a few years prior. What descended upon us was not just a novel virus but a novel mode of social organization and control. The bureaucratic phrase for this was stay-at-home orders, but the public embraced the more apt term: lockdowns.

This term originated not in medicine or public health but the penal system. Prisons go into lockdown to restore order when prisoners riot. When the most tightly controlled and surveilled environment on the planet erupts into chaos, order is restored by asserting swift and complete control of the entire prison population by force. Only strictly surveilled confinement can keep the dangerous and unruly population in check. Prisoners cannot be permitted to riot; inmates cannot run the asylum.

In February of 2020, our society believed that chaos was coming, and we embraced the idea that this penal solution was the right, indeed the only sensible, response. Lockdowns met remarkably little resistance when initially implemented. Fifteen days to flatten the curve seemed reasonable to most people. This would buy a bit of time for us to gain a handle on the new virus, get our bearings, and prevent loved ones from dying in the streets because hospitals were overrun with patients.

One after another in rapid succession, state governors ordered us to stay at home. We readily obeyed. To refuse, we were told, was to recklessly court death. Any small pockets of resistance were swiftly stigmatized. As one journalist described it, "Appeals to science were weaponized to enforce conformity, and the media portrayed anti-lockdown protesters as backwards, astroturfed white nationalists bent on endangering the public."[28] Who wanted to be classed in that camp?

Reports about covid had already mesmerized the world for a few months leading up to lockdowns. We stayed glued to screens, watching case counts rise as we tracked coronavirus deaths in foreign countries. Social media exploded with scary images from Northern Italy, where hospitals struggled under severe strain and panicked emergency room doctors warned that this wave of disease and death would soon hit our shores. The media failed to mention that the health care system in this region of an ostensibly first-world country had been for years severely compromised and underfunded, or that these hospitals in Lombardy had been routinely overwhelmed for the last several years during seasonal influenza outbreaks.

Not yet seeing our own cases in the United States and the United Kingdom, we relied for guidance on mathematical modeling. Because we were primed for panic, the model chosen was not one of the many sober statistical predictions, but the terrifying numbers published by Neil Ferguson's group at the Imperial College in London, which predicted 40 million deaths by May 2020. We conveniently ignored Ferguson's dismal track record of wildly overestimated predictions in prior epidemics, and we sidelined critics like the legendary biostatistician John Ioannidis of Stanford, who warned that the Imperial College model was grounded in seriously faulty assumptions.

No matter, this time, surely, Ferguson's dire prophesies would be vindicated. As it turned out, this model was proven more wildly wrong than any of the other leading models on offer. The Imperial College model predicted that if it did not lock down, Sweden would have 80,000 deaths by the end of May. It remained one of the few countries that did not lock down and had 6,000 deaths, even using methods resulting in overcounting. Ferguson's model was testable and was clearly proven wrong by May 2020, though that fact did nothing to shift our trajectory.[29]

In the earliest months of the pandemic, I spent nights and weekends knee-deep in worst-case-scenario planning, helping the University of California draft its pandemic triage policies. In 2020 I was a clinical professor at the University of California, Irvine, School of Medicine and director of the Medical Ethics Program at UCI Health, where I had spent my entire fifteen-year career. I joined with critical care specialists and bioethicists from the other four UC hospitals on a workgroup convened by the UC Office of the President, which oversaw all the branch campuses. Our first task was to devise crisis standards of care: a ventilator triage policy that would have been applied if the demand for ventilators outstripped our supply.

The ethical questions we wrestled with were not purely academic: many of us believed this policy might need to be implemented at our institutions in a matter of weeks or months, and we were working against the clock to prepare. Hospitals in New York were reporting that, if help did not come, they might run out of ventilators. The West Coast surely would not have to wait long for our own covid nightmare, we thought. Most of the committee members were frontline physicians with skin in the game. In an article I wrote at the time, "The Impossible Ethics of Pandemic Triage," I reflected on the experience:

> We have deliberated about duty, justice, equality, fairness, transparency. These principles can never be abandoned even in a crisis. Yet something lingers always in the background of our efforts. There is an inescapably tragic undercurrent to all of this, however upright our intentions. This one unsettling fact always remains to haunt us: If hospitals exceed their surge capacity, patients who otherwise would have lived will die. Lives will be lost simply because we lacked the resources to offer everyone the basics of modern medicine.
>
> T. S. Eliot saw the limits of our ability to rectify all wrongs and balance the scales of justice when he wrote, "For us, there is only the trying. The rest is not our business." My colleagues and I, like so many others in these strange times, are trying our best. But controlling and managing this pandemic is beyond our abilities, indeed, beyond anyone's abilities. In the absence of a God's-eye view, in the absence of unlimited resources, in the absence of a crystal ball that can perfectly prognosticate outcomes, physicians are left to do whatever we can—even as we know that this will not be enough. For us there is only the trying. The rest is marked by tragedy.[30]

I now see that the tragic sense I wrote about here was prescient, but not for the reasons I imagined then. With worries of an impending disaster, I initially supported "two weeks of lockdowns to flatten the curve." California became one of the first states to implement a statewide stay-at-home order to prevent the worst-case scenario we had been preparing for, supposedly to avoid overwhelming our health care system. Or so I thought at the time.

• • •

The first days of lockdown felt surreal. While nearly everyone stayed at home, I donned my scrubs and drove to the hospital every day. The stretch of Interstate 5 between my house in San Juan Capistrano and the hospital twenty-five miles north in Orange was typically thick with morning traffic. But during lockdowns I drove long stretches of this road at eighty miles an hour without a single car in sight. The Southern California smog cleared after a week or two, and the sunny sky turned a richer blue. In a hunch that turned out to be right, I recall thinking at the time, "When this is over, they're going to propose lockdowns to deal with climate change."

Before the end of the year, we saw policy analysts floating this proposal. For example, Mariana Mazzucato, author of *The Entrepreneurial State* and professor at University College London, wrote in September 2020 that—absent a complete overhaul in our economic systems—climate lockdowns would soon be necessary to avoid disaster: "Under a 'climate lockdown,' governments would limit private-vehicle use, ban consumption of red meat, and impose extreme energy-saving measures, while fossil-fuel companies would have to stop drilling."

One might have thought that covid and climate change were distinct issues, but she explained that "COVID-19 is itself a consequence of environmental degradation. . . . Moreover, climate change will exacerbate the social and economic problems highlighted by the pandemic." Therefore, she concludes, "The climate crisis is also a public-health crisis."[31] We were not yet through one crisis before policy wonks were anticipating the use of lockdowns for the next one, redefining an environmental issue as a public health problem.

But in March 2020, the lockdowns were still about covid, or so I assumed. While everything else in sight—businesses, restaurants, food trucks—lay fallow and dormant, I expected to arrive at a hospital still buzzing with the usual activity. To my surprise, the hospital wards were likewise eerily empty, without visitors, but also with very few patients. For a week or two we figured this must be the calm before the storm. We waited. Two weeks stretched into three, then four; March slid into April. The lockdowns continued but the hospital remained quiet. The long-anticipated surge was surely coming; the tsunami was no doubt still just a few miles offshore. May came, and still nothing. All quiet on the Western front. Although covid hospital admissions eventually rose that summer, we had waited for an overwhelming surge that never arrived.

Fear of the virus, stoked by around-the-clock news reports tracking case counts and covid deaths, scared away people with other conditions from seeking care in emergency rooms and clinics. Aside from the drop in motor-vehicle accident victims in the trauma bay of the ER, it was not that the usual patients were any healthier. It was simply that the sick stayed away. People feared that hospitals with covid patients would be more dangerous to their health than forgoing surgeries or declining care. Our clinics were so dry and deserted in the early months of the pandemic that many doctors and nurses were sent home on furlough. Nationwide, "1.4 million hospital staff were laid off during lockdowns" in April of 2020, "while private health insurance companies doubled their earnings" on money they had not spent on patient care.[32] Meanwhile, the sick cowered at home in fear, and the chronically ill languished without care.

Within weeks I could see the harms of lockdowns manifesting in the patients I treated in our psychiatric clinic. Their outlook was apocalyptic; many were frozen with terror. I recall one middle-aged woman we saw in the resident clinic I supervised. She was consuming hours of CNN daily. This patient was neither psychotic nor manic, neither paranoid nor delusional. Yet she literally thought the end of the world was nigh. When I suggested she turn off the television news for a bit, since it was clearly harming her mental health, she told me she feared missing something important. I suggested that, whether she watched the news or not, if the president was assassinated, she would hear about it. "That's not what I worry about," she replied, "in fact, I hope that happens." I was not sure how to respond to that.

This patient was not alone: people of all political persuasions were speaking in these apocalyptic tones, paralyzed with fear and willing to do anything to escape the impending viral doom. Even so, the end-of-the-world mathematical models were proven dead wrong: doomsday never arrived. When the first covid wave finally came in the summer of 2020, our hospital and the others in California came nowhere near exceeding our surge capacity. A navy field-hospital ship docked in Los Angeles harbor was never used. The first floor of our psychiatry building was converted to accommodate covid patients, but those beds remained empty throughout the pandemic.

After briefly loosening lockdown restrictions, cases started to rise again that summer and the governor ordered the lockdowns to resume. The UC hospitals were only at 10 to 20 percent ventilator occupancy—nowhere near our maximum surge capacity—when Governor Newsom reinstated lockdowns. By then I was long since disillusioned with the lockdown strategy. I could not fathom why our government was doing this. Rolling lockdowns were not necessary to avoid hospital triage. That lockdowns failed to stop the spread of covid became clearer with each passing month. Lockdowns succeeded only in fostering a sense of perpetual crisis.

After the first month, nobody spoke of flattening the curve anymore. When the new mantra became "stay home to save lives," the stated rationale for lockdowns involved systematic mendacity and carefully couched half-truths. Distancing could not save lives in the aggregate, but at best slow the spread temporarily. For a respiratory virus pandemic to end, we needed herd immunity. There are only two ways to get that: a highly effective and safe vaccine that prevents infection and transmission of the virus, or a sufficient proportion of the population infected who thereby acquire natural immunity, or some combination of those two. Anything else was just dragging out the inevitable. I could not understand why the immunologists and epidemiologists remained silent about these basic facts during the lockdowns—facts that every first-year medical student should have clearly understood.

More than just an unjustified assault on civil liberties, lockdowns were an ineffectual public health measure: they failed to achieve their own stated aims. In January 2022 scholars at the Johns Hopkins Institute for Applied Economics, Global Health, and the Study of Business Enterprise published "A Literature Review and Meta-Analysis of the Effects of Lockdowns on COVID-19 Mortality."[33] In scientific publications a systematic review provides a qualitative summary of the findings of several studies, chosen for their methodological rigor according to strict inclusion criteria. A meta-analysis pools data from several smaller studies to present a quantitative synthesis of their findings. This is one way to overcome some of the limitations of each individual study, and the findings of a good meta-analysis are often invaluable.

The Johns Hopkins researchers conducted both types of analysis and concluded: "Lockdowns have had little to no effect on COVID-19 mortality. More specifically, stringency index studies find that lockdowns in Europe and the United States only reduced COVID-19 mortality by 0.2% on average." The authors also summarize the findings regarding collateral harms: "While this meta-analysis concludes that lockdowns have had little to no public health effects, they have imposed enormous economic and social costs where they have been adopted." The researchers therefore conclude, "In consequence, lockdown policies are ill-founded and should be rejected as a pandemic policy instrument.[34]

The damage inflicted by our failed lockdowns and school closure policies is impossible to calculate and will be felt for decades. Despite this there is now talk in the air of another lockdown. Recently, the British government advised citizens to work from home three days a week to deal with the oil crisis created by Russia's invasion of Ukraine. It seems likely that, despite the failures of this method of social control, lockdowns will be deployed again during the next declared public health crisis or the next state of emergency. Rejecting this failed policy will require understanding and dismantling the biosecurity paradigm of which lockdowns form an essential part.

● ● ●

Tocqueville warned us that democracy contains built-in vulnerabilities that can lead democratic nations to deteriorate into despotism. New levels of political irresponsibility came when we took a totalitarian state as the model for managing a pandemic. Recall that China was the birthplace of lockdowns. The first state-ordered lockdown occurred in Wuhan and nearby Chinese cities. In mid-February 2020, the WHO sent a delegation to China, which included, among other NIH employees, Clifford Lane, Anthony Fauci's deputy at the NIAID division of NIH.

Three days later the delegation published its *Report of the WHO-China Joint Mission on Coronavirus Disease 2019 (COVID-19)* which praised China's strategy: "China's uncompromising and rigorous use of non-pharmaceutical measures [lockdowns] to contain transmission of the COVID-19 virus in multiple settings provides vital lessons for the global response. This rather unique and unprecedented public health response in China reversed the escalating cases," the report claimed.[35] My colleague Jeffrey Tucker at the Brownstone Institute gave a tongue-in-cheek gloss of WHO's misty-eyed report: "We have seen the future. It is Wuhan."[36]

Lockdowns quickly spread from China to the West, as a troubling number of Western apologists besides the WHO also looked to the Chinese Communist Party's covid response for guidance. The CCP advertised that they had stamped out the virus in the regions where they had locked down. This was clearly false advertising, but the WHO and most nations bought it. The United States and the United Kingdom followed Italy's lockdown, which had followed China, and all but a handful of countries around the globe immediately followed our lead.[37] Within weeks the whole world was locked down.

The World Health Organization was established in 1948 as the health-policy body within the United Nations and was given the mission to "direct and coordinate the world's response to health emergencies."[38] Its mission since then has become hopelessly compromised by strong reliance on funding from China and from private benefactors. Today, Bill Gates's foundation funds 13 percent of the WHO budget—more than any other private contributor, indeed, more than any other government except the United States. In the early days of the pandemic, the WHO was slow to call for a comprehensive investigation on the origins of the virus.[39] The WHO's director general, echoing the delegation's report, praised the early 2020 lockdowns in Wuhan. In a January 2020 letter, the WHO congratulated China on its covid measures and urged the CCP to "enhance public health measures for containment of the current outbreak."[40]

WHO director general Tedros Adhanom Ghebreyesus, speaking like a wholly owned subsidiary of the CCP, punctuated this letter with a tweet: "In many ways, #China is actually setting a new standard of outbreak response. Our greatest concern is the potential for the virus to spread to countries with weaker health systems, and which are ill-prepared to deal with it."[41] Neil Ferguson, mastermind of the apocalyptic Imperial College London predictions, likewise looked to China as a model: "It's a communist one party state, we said. We couldn't get away with it [locking down] in Europe, we thought . . . and then Italy did it. And we realized we could."[42] Considering Ferguson's remarks, it's perhaps not coincidental that when President Xi Jinping of the People's Republic of China visited Imperial College London in October 2015, the college's president Alice Gast effused, "Imperial College London strives to be China's best academic partner in the West." Cutting edge research collaborations between Imperial College and the Chinese has included work in public health.[43]

Communist regimes always reconceptualize nature, including human nature, as an artificial system. They then attempt to control this system as though it is nothing but an inert mechanistic mass. This is among the reasons that communist ideologies inevitably fail when they encounter systems that will not bend to their ideological will but continue to operate according to the laws of nature. In April 2022, as happened the previous month in South Korea, the bills from the Chinese zero-covid strategy, which followed this disastrous template, came due.

The Chinese Communist Party's continued adherence to this ideology led to a nightmare scene, symbolized by the city of Shanghai's draconian lockdowns. The Western media mostly looked away while the city descended into a hellscape. Jeffrey Tucker described the situation in Shanghai, which had initiated a *totalizing* lockdown as covid cases rose: "Children are being taken from parents, the pets of people with a positive test are being shot, people are screaming from skyscrapers, and food is rotting in warehouses even as people report to be starving," he described. "There are videos online of stores being ransacked. There is talk of revolution in the air."[44]

A Bloomberg article on April 7 likewise painted a gruesome picture of Shanghai during this maniacal police-state enforced lockdown: "Pets beaten to death. Parents forced to separate from their children. Elderly folks unable to access medical care. Locked-up residents chanting 'we want to eat' and 'we want freedom.'" Shanghai resident Lily Chen told a reporter, "In this country it's not the virus that scares us, but the chaotic anti-Covid measures that have caused risks to the well-being of the elderly, the children and companion animals." She concluded, "I now realize we can only rely on ourselves—not the government—to protect our own families."[45]

Residents of the city complained on social media about running out of food, cancer medications, and baby formula. The government's lockdown regulations and failure to supply food left one mother "skipping meals" to make sure her parents and children had enough to eat. "I cannot cook because we have nothing to cook," she explained. Radio France Internationale reported that a "44-year-old Korean man living in Shanghai was found dead in his apartment"; the lockdown deprived him of cardiac medications he needed to treat a heart problem. Shanghai's twenty thousand patients requiring routine dialysis could not access this life-sustaining treatment.[46]

Videos shared on social media showed "government employees in hazmat suits erecting fences to keep people caged in their residences." While locked in their apartment buildings, to overcome their loneliness people opened windows to sing together and "chant that they were hungry." Some, overcome by grief from the extreme isolation, were seen jumping to their deaths. The CCP sent out drones with loudspeakers that blared prerecorded messages on repeat: "Control your soul's desire for freedom. Do not open the window or sing."[47]

Two years of China's zero-covid lockdown ideology had prepared a tinderbox in Shanghai. Instead of a slow-burn spread of the virus over time, resulting in a population with significant natural immunity, omicron hit a vulnerable covid-naïve population armed only with leaky vaccines. Despite its totalitarian-level lockdowns, daily cases in Shanghai skyrocketed to twenty-one thousand and China's health care system was overrun with patients.[48]

In a horror movie story so shocking it would be unbelievable if not verified on film, CNBC reported that an elderly man mistaken for dead was transported from his nursing home to the morgue in a hearse. When health workers in blue-and-white protective gear pulled the body bag out of the car, one of them shouted, "He's alive!" Although the man was eventually returned to his nursing home, if he had not stirred at that moment, his weakened body would have been incinerated with the corpses.[49]

As a physician friend who is a professor at Stanford likes to say, nature always bats in the bottom of the ninth inning. And nature is never subject to our complete control, even in a totalitarian state. The virus is gonna virus. By April of 2022, and likely well before this, there was no doubt the Chinese authorities knew that lockdowns could not stop the omicron variant. Zero covid was a pretense for a political crackdown. A quiet movement of citizens leaving the Chinese Communist Party had been afoot for more than a year, and Shanghai with its international flair was among the nodes of resistance. The lockdown of 2022 was doubtless political theater, for even hardboiled communists know that health cannot be a justification for moving from biomedical security to biomedical terror.

During the Shanghai lockdowns, videos surfaced of Chinese authorities disinfecting roads. Workers donning full-body hazmat suits and industrial-grade respirators straddled a frontloading tractor, shoveling white powder onto the street and dusting up a hazy white cloud in their wake.[50] Someone looking out the window and seeing this pass by their yard might wonder whether this was caustic lye or just talcum powder used for theatrical effect. No matter, the visual image of biosecurity terror was the same. In this regime the brownshirts and blackshirts had exchanged their uniforms for hazmat suits of sterile white and hospital blue.

Because, after all, lockdowns are about public health.

The Other Pandemic

Two weeks to flatten the curve stretched into endless months of lockdowns. By October of 2020, I could see the giant shipping barges stacked and parked offshore as I drove along the Pacific Coast Highway near my home. The ports of Los Angeles and Long Beach, which handle 40 percent of all U.S. container imports, were suffering from a shortage of workers, from truck drivers to mechanics. Long Beach became ground zero of the United States' months-long supply chain crisis. At that time there were seventy-six ships—ninety-three if we include the ones further offshore that were also in the queue—waiting at the Long Beach Port, with 430,000 containers full of goods worth $26 billion. Only seven out of hundreds of the port's cranes were operating, and less than a dozen containers were unloaded daily. The port was short around four thousand truckers, further exacerbating the backlog.[51]

Government, with cooperation from the media, tried to conceal from the public the stark realities of our lockdown policies by making the ships park further offshore, over the horizon, so they could not be seen. This political strategy of addressing a problem by removing it from sight is a useful metaphor for most other aspects of our covid response. The supply chain crisis created by lockdowns and exacerbated by vaccine mandates became increasingly difficult to hide over time: by June 2022, the *Washington Post* reported an alarming months-long national shortage of baby formula in the United States. "According to the retail analysis firm Datasembly, starting the week of April 24," the *Post* reported, "the amount of formula available on shelves was 40 percent below normal inventory levels. . . . In several states, there is half as much formula on shelves as customers would normally expect."[52] Baby formula shortages—in the world's wealthiest country.

The supply chain crisis was by no means the worst effect of the lockdowns. After a few months of lockdowns, my early concern about collateral harms of this policy escalated to alarm that we were ignoring the real crisis. I published an article in October 2021 titled "The Other Pandemic," which described the mental health crisis—a crisis created not by the virus but by our response to the virus. The problems I was treating in clinic were by then confirmed by solid research.

But these findings received little attention from the public health establishment and our governing authorities, who continued to focus exclusively on covid case counts. Public health—which was supposed to be about the health of the population as a whole and not just one disease—was willingly conscripted in interstate rivalries between governors focused exclusively on bringing down covid metrics. I wrote then about the tight link between lockdown policies and the anticipated hope for a vaccine that would end the pandemic:

> The political rhetoric now suggests we are "saving lives" by continuing to keep people at home. But locking down alone does not in the end save lives; it only slows the spread of the virus. The (usually unspoken) hope of politicians is that we can do this until we have an effective vaccine. That is an enormous gamble based on an axiological faith in science to solve our problems, which cannot be justified scientifically.

After all, it is plausible that scientists created this virus in a lab in the first place—a claim no longer in the realm of conspiracy theory.[53]

When the vaccines were first released, this gamble seemed to have paid off. But as it turned out, the questions I raised in October 2020 about the vaccine gambit were prescient:

> The reason that public messaging now involves dishonesty is that locking down to "save lives" really means "stay locked down until we have an effective vaccine and sufficient time to distribute that vaccine to the population.". . . The threshold the FDA has set for approving a vaccine for covid is that it needs to be 50 percent more effective than placebo at preventing disease (note: not at preventing *transmission*). This is roughly what we get from the annual flu vaccine. Let's suppose the initial vaccines meet that threshold. Will 50 percent efficacy be sufficient to end the lockdowns? If not, do we continue with this until we get a better vaccine? Again, if we end up with a partially effective vaccine—a likely scenario—we will still be left with another series of questions that no politician wants to answer. It is easier to stick to the simplistic meme, "stay home to save lives" and hope that people don't ask any pointed questions.[54]

Regardless of how the vaccine gamble eventually turned out, the mental health harms of lockdowns were by then evident. By summer of 2020 nearly half of Americans reported the coronavirus crisis was harming their mental health. We would expect a pandemic of this magnitude to adversely impact our mental health. But the duration and magnitude of the mental health crisis was not inevitable. It was mostly a problem of our own creation, a problem created by our lockdown policies and school closures.

In August 2020 the CDC published a devastating report on the mental health effects of lockdowns, from a population-based survey in June of over five thousand Americans. Four out of ten respondents reported at least one adverse mental or behavioral health condition. Three out of ten reported symptoms of anxiety disorder or depressive disorder, and one-quarter reported symptoms of a trauma- or stressor-related disorder due to the pandemic, such as PTSD. Thirteen percent reported having started or increased substance use to cope with stress or emotions related to covid lockdowns.

Of particular concern, 11 percent reported they had seriously contemplated suicide in the past thirty days. Among eighteen-to-twenty-four-year-olds, this number was 25 percent. We should pause to consider this finding: one-quarter of young adults in America contemplated suicide during lockdowns in June 2020. Rates of suicidal thinking that month were higher among minorities (Hispanic 19 percent, black 15 percent), among unpaid caregivers for adults (31 percent), and essential workers (22 percent). Compared to June 2019, one year prior, prevalence of anxiety disorders had tripled (26 percent versus 8 percent), and prevalence of depressive disorders had quadrupled (24 percent versus 6 percent). These were extremely sobering statistics: it is exceptionally rare to see these kinds of shifts in psychiatric epidemiology from one year to the next.[55]

Military officials argued in September 2020 that social distancing rules and the pressures of lockdowns were contributing to the 20 percent rise in suicides among U.S. military service members that year. But nobody listened. We knew that "deaths of despair" (that is, suicide, drug-overdose, and alcohol-related deaths) were on the rise prior to the pandemic, and the opioid crisis was already taking a massive toll. Against this backdrop we saw sharp increases in opioid-overdose deaths during the lockdowns, with more than forty states recording increases in opioid-related deaths in 2020.[56]

The opioid crisis—the worse drug crisis in U.S. history—fueled an enormous rise in deaths by drug overdose even prior to the pandemic, rising from less than twenty thousand in the year 2000 to seventy thousand by 2019. Lockdowns poured gasoline on that fire: in 2021 the number of deaths by drug overdose rose 29 percent to one hundred thousand. This number was rarely reported by the media alongside covid statistics.[57]

Alcohol-related deaths similarly increased 25 percent during the first year of lockdowns, reaching ninety-nine thousand in 2020, up from seventy-nine thousand the previous year, according to an NIH study published in the *Journal of the American Medical Association*. The largest increases occurred in people from thirty-five to forty-four years old (40 percent increase) and people from twenty-five to thirty-four years old (37 percent increase).[58] In Japan during October 2020, suicide accounted for more deaths in one month than covid had killed that entire year.[59]

Lockdowns had other adverse effects on the very population they were meant to protect, namely, the elderly. A September 2020 analysis of CDC data by the *Washington Post* found about 13,200 excess deaths due to Alzheimer's and other forms of dementia since lockdowns began in March that year. According to the article:

> People with dementia are dying not just from the virus but from the very strategy of isolation that's supposed to protect them. In recent months, doctors have reported increased falls, pulmonary infections, depression and sudden frailty in patients who had been stable for years. Social and mental stimulation are among the few tools that can slow the march of dementia.[60]

We already knew that social isolation could kill. Loneliness and social fragmentation were epidemic even prior to the coronavirus pandemic. As Nobel Prize–winning Princeton researchers Ann Case and Angus Deaton had demonstrated, these factors were contributing to rising rates of deaths of despair. Since the 1980s, reported loneliness among adults in the United States increased from 20 percent to 40 percent.[61] In this context, consider the "Alone Together" public service announcement produced for the government by the Ad Council in March of 2020. The ad read, "Staying home saves lives. Whether you have COVID-19 or not, stay home! We'll be here to keep you company. #AloneTogether."[62] The very conjunction of these two words, a manifest contradiction, is enough to demonstrate the absurdity.

It is no accident that one of the most severe punishments we inflict on prisoners is solitary confinement—a condition that eventually leads to sensory disintegration and psychosis. During lockdowns we embraced and actively promoted what philosopher Hannah Arendt called "organized loneliness," a social state she identified as a precondition for totalitarianism in her seminal book *The Origins of Totalitarianism*.[63]

The carnage was not, as many news reports misleadingly suggested, collateral damage inflicted by *coronavirus*. No, this was collateral damage inflicted by our *policy response* to covid, especially by the deeply misguided and ineffective lockdown strategy. The authors of the study cited above on alcohol-related deaths in 2020 noted, for example, that "only a small proportion of the increase in alcohol-related deaths involved COVID-19 directly."[64] Our collective policy decisions, not the virus, created the toxic social conditions that increased the deaths of despair. In contrast to covid deaths, the young were disproportionately impacted by "The Other Pandemic."

● ● ●

As the chair of our hospital's medical ethics committee, I had more conversations than I can count with family members whose loved ones were irretrievably dying of covid in our hospital. Our committee was consulted routinely to assist with these difficult conversations. One of the worst moments for me during the pandemic came during one of these family meetings in early 2020.

I was speaking to the wife and son of a man dying of covid. After extensive explanation and discussion of the dire medical situation, the family agreed to transition him to comfort care only. Naturally, this was an anguishing decision, but they wisely wanted to avoid unnecessarily prolonging the dying process by burdening him with additional ineffective interventions. The family then asked us for assistance in making funeral arrangements. They were from Mexico, did not speak English, had little money, and needed the hospital social worker to help them navigate this.

To my horror the social worker informed them that because the patient had covid, the hospital (following the CDC's recommendation) would not return the body to the family for burial. Instead, his remains would be cremated without the patient's or family's consent. The family explained that the patient was Catholic and would have wanted a traditional Christian burial. They felt duty-bound to honor his wish. The public health authority's insistence on cremation was based upon an entirely theoretical and facially absurd risk that, just perhaps, a corpse could still spread covid. It mattered little that there was not one shred of evidence for this notion from previous respiratory viruses. This idea was eventually disproven, of course, but by then thousands of families had endured the loss of the right to bury their loved one.

I was struck then by a pattern I continued to see during the pandemic: a *real, known, present* human good, a familial and spiritual good—burying the dead, in this case—was sacrificed on the altar of a *theoretical, unknown, future* biological risk. It was obvious we were harming the family by this refusal; yet the mere potential for some type of medical risk, a potential that was in fact scientifically groundless, trumped this clear and present harm.

This was the biosecurity paradigm of governance at work. I was dumbstruck by this manifestation of our new sanitary terror. Many recall that we were not permitted to attend funerals during lockdowns, and this was bad enough. Fewer are aware that for several months people were not permitted to bury their loved ones at all, whether they could attend the funeral service or not. Not since the time of Antigone had Western nations forbidden citizens to bury the dead.

Kheriaty versus the University of California

Shortly after I published the *Wall Street Journal* piece arguing that university vaccine mandates were unethical, the University of California, my employer, promulgated its vaccine mandate. I decided then it was time to put a stake in the ground: I filed lawsuit in federal court challenging the constitutionality of the university's vaccine mandate on behalf of covid-recovered individuals. It was already clear from many robust studies that natural immunity following infection was superior to vaccine-mediated immunity in terms of efficacy and duration of immunity.

Thus, forcing those like me with natural immunity to be vaccinated introduced unnecessary risks without commensurate benefits—either to individuals or to the population as a whole—and violated our equal protection rights guaranteed under the Constitution's Fourteenth Amendment. Expert-witness documents in support of my case included a declaration from distinguished UCLA and UCSF School of Medicine faculty members and other luminaries, such as Dr. Peter McCullough, Dr. Joseph Ladapo, who was then at UCLA but later that year was appointed Surgeon General of Florida, and Dr. Aditi Bhargava of University of California, San Francisco.

At the time I was an unlikely candidate to challenge the prevailing vaccination policies. I was deeply embedded in the academic medical establishment, where I had spent my entire career. In my capacity as a psychiatric consultant on the medical wards and in the emergency department, I had suited up in PPE (personal protective equipment) to see hundreds of hospitalized covid patients, witnessing the worst that this illness can do. Nobody needed to explain to me how bad this virus could be for some individuals, especially the elderly with co-occurring medical conditions who were at significant risk of bad outcomes when infected.

I contracted the virus in July 2020, and despite my efforts to self-isolate, passed it to my wife and five children. Living and breathing covid for a year, I eagerly awaited a safe and effective vaccine for those that were still not immune to this virus. I happily served on the Orange County COVID-19 Vaccine Task Force, and I advocated in the *Los*

Angeles Times that the elderly and sick be prioritized for vaccination, and that the poor, disabled, and underserved be given ready access to vaccines.[65]

I had worked every day for over a year to develop and advance the university's and state's pandemic mitigation measures. But as the prevailing covid policies unfolded, I became increasingly concerned, and eventually disillusioned. Our one-size-fits-all coercive mandates failed to take account of individualized risks and benefits, particularly age-stratified risks, which are central to the practice of good medicine. We ignored foundational principles of public health, like transparency and the health of the entire population. With little resistance we abandoned foundational ethical principles.

Among the most glaring failures of our response to covid was the refusal to acknowledge the natural immunity of covid-recovered patients in our mitigation strategies, herd-immunity estimates, and vaccine-rollout plans. The CDC estimated that by May 2021, more than 120 million Americans (36 percent) had been infected with covid. Following the delta-variant wave later that year, many epidemiologists estimated the number was close to half of all Americans. By the end of omicron wave in early 2022, that number was north of 70 percent.[66] The good news—almost never mentioned—was that those with previous infection had more durable and longer lasting immunity than the vaccinated. Yet the focus remained exclusively on vaccines.

The largest population-based study comparing natural immunity to vaccine immunity found that fully vaccinated individuals were six to thirteen times more likely to get infected than previously infected unvaccinated individuals. The risk of developing symptomatic covid was twenty-seven times higher among the vaccinated compared to previously infected, and the risk of hospitalization was eight times higher.[67] These findings were not surprising, since infection with the virus allows our body to form a broad and diverse immune response to many parts (antigens) on the virus, whereas the vaccines expose us only to one part, the spike protein. Furthermore, evidence from several studies found that covid-recovered individuals were at higher risk of vaccine-adverse effects compared to those not previously infected.[68]

As I argued in a coauthored article, medical exemptions for most vaccine mandates were too narrowly tailored, constraining physician's discretionary judgment and seriously compromising individualized patient care.[69] Most mandates only allowed medical exemptions for conditions included on the CDC's list of contraindications to the vaccines—a list that was never meant to be comprehensive. CDC recommendations should never have been taken as sound medical advice applicable to every patient. My coauthors and I explained the problems with treating the CDC as a kind of "super-doctor" for the entire nation:

> The CDC is not a medical institution; it is a public health and disease prevention body. According to the CDC's own mission statement, the agency focuses on "disease prevention and control, environmental health, and health promotion and health education activities." It is not qualified and usually does not purport to offer professional medical opinions applicable to specific patients. From time to time, the CDC offers findings and recommendations that competent medical practitioners often will consider in arriving at a professional medical judgment for a particular patient. In this respect, CDC guidelines are analogous to guidelines from other public health associations or medical societies: they are *guidelines*, not prescriptions.[70]

Further exacerbating this problem, on August 17, 2021, all licensed physicians in California received a notification from the state medical board with the heading "Inappropriate Exemptions May Subject Physicians to Discipline." Physicians were informed that any doctor granting an inappropriate mask exemption or other covid-related exemptions "may be subjecting their license to disciplinary action." In what was perhaps a deliberate omission, the "standard of care" criteria for vaccine exemptions was never defined by the medical board. In my eighteen years as a licensed physician, I had never previously received any such notice, nor had my colleagues.

The effect was chilling: since physicians naturally interpreted "other exemptions" to include vaccines, it became de facto impossible to find a doctor in California willing to write a medical exemption, even if the patient had a legitimate contraindication to the covid vaccines. One of my patients was told by his rheumatologist he should not get the covid vaccine, since he was at low risk from covid and in this physician's judgment his autoimmune condition elevated his risks of vaccine adverse effects. This patient, who was subjected to a vaccine mandate at work, immediately asked this same physician for a medical exemption. The doctor replied, "I'm sorry, I cannot write you an exemption because I'm afraid I might lose my license." I heard many stories of similar egregious violations of medical ethics under these repressive mandates and the enforcement regime that bolstered them.

Even as it became clear that vaccine efficacy was waning with time and new variants—and that serious safety signals of adverse vaccine reactions were emerging, especially in young people—public and private institutions nevertheless ramped up their efforts to coercively mandate universal vaccination. In justifying these mandates, officials elided the huge gulf between the following claims: (1) that one can make a plausible public health argument that everyone should be vaccinated, and (2) we can and should coerce everyone to be vaccinated. The second claim in no way followed necessarily from the first.

As the vaccines rolled out in 2021, I spoke to many students, faculty, residents, staff, and patients who were aware of these basic immunological facts and were asking legitimate questions about vaccine mandates. Many correctly saw no medical or public health justification for subjecting themselves to the risks of the novel vaccines when they already had superior natural immunity. Others had moral concerns but did not qualify for a religious exemption, because religion was not central to their conscience-based objections.

They felt intimidated, disempowered, and vulnerable in the face of immense pressure to go along. Many physicians and nurses were afraid to speak up in the climate of coercion. Public health officials ignored inconvenient scientific findings, suppressed reasonable questions, and bullied into silence any skeptical physicians or scientists. Institutions promulgating mandates stigmatized and punished those who refused to comply. I had never seen anything like this in medicine.

The manipulation of language became so pervasive and habitual during the mass vaccination campaign that authorities didn't blink when stating blatant contradictions. For example, the University of California's medical portal for staff contained a box employees had to "voluntarily" check in our medical record to release covid vaccine information under the UC mandate. The following two adjacent lines on the required form perfectly expressed the obvious contradiction with the juxtaposition of the words "mandate" and "consent":

UC Covid-19 Vaccine Mandate
[ ] Consent to share Covid vaccine information

Why did I file a lawsuit in federal court against my own employer? I had nothing to gain personally by this and a lot to lose professionally. I decided I could not stand by and watch the ethical disaster unfold around me without attempting to do something. In my position as Director of Medical Ethics at UCI, I had a duty to represent those whose voices were silenced and to insist upon the right of informed consent and informed refusal.

In the end, my decision to challenge these mandates came down to this question: How could I continue to call myself a medical ethicist if I failed to do what I was convinced was morally right under pressure? Projecting ahead to the required medical ethics course I taught to first- and second-year medical students at the beginning of each year, I could not imagine lecturing on informed consent, moral courage, and our duty to protect patients from harm if I had failed to oppose these unjust and unscientific mandates. I simply would not have woken up each day with a clear conscience.

● ● ●

The university did not take kindly to my legal challenge, as you might imagine. Administrators allowed no grass to grow under their feet before responding to this dissident within the ranks. I had petitioned the court for a preliminary injunction to put the vaccine mandate on hold while the case was litigated in court. The judge declined this request, and the following day the university placed me on "investigatory leave" for alleged noncompliance with the vaccine mandate. Instead of waiting for the federal court to decide my case, the university immediately banned me from working on campus or working from home.

I was given no opportunity to contact my patients, students, residents, or colleagues and let them know I would suddenly disappear. An email from one of the deans, sent after I had left the office for the day, informed me that I could not return to campus the following day. As I drove away from campus for the last time that day, I glanced at the sign on the corner near the hospital. The sign, which had been up for months, read in large block letters, HEROES WORK HERE.

That same day, as it happened, I received a university-wide email sent to all campus employees: "The Office of the President has invited comments on a proposed Presidential Policy on Abusive Conduct/Bullying in the Workplace. The proposed policy covers abusive conduct/bullying and retaliation by and against members of the University community in the workplace." Oh, okay.

A month later the university placed me on unpaid suspension and forbade me to see my patients. In violation of every principle of fair employment, the university also tried to prevent me from doing any outside professional activities while I was on unpaid suspension. The associate dean later admitted under oath, during an academic senate hearing to appeal the decision, that I was the only faculty member they ever specifically instructed not to engage in other professional activities while suspended without pay.

The administration also refused to allow me to take my accrued nine weeks of paid time off, which would have provided an income to support my family during this period of suspension. To pressure me to resign, the university attempted to entirely hamstring my ability to earn any income. The ordeal was dizzying and at times surreal. I could not work because I was not vaccinated; and I could not stay at home on vacation because . . . I was not vaccinated. All in the name of . . . science!

I was one of countless thousands who suffered a similar fate under coercive vaccine mandates that year. Shortly after I was suspended, I received the following in an email from a fellow UCI professor—a progressive man of the Left—who was supportive of my lawsuit and sympathetic to my situation. His remarks, included here with his permission, illustrate the climate of fear and coercion that were operative in countless institutions under the vaccine mandate regime:

> I have felt completely silenced given the large-scale, CDC, media, and now UC Regents driven demonization of anyone daring to offer critical questions with respect to the exclusion of the category of natural immunity from conversations about the pandemic and best practices in that regard. I am [a] Black person, on a single-income, and remain basically one lost paycheck away from economic precarity so I have felt pressured into remaining silent on this issue given the way those who have spoken out have been attacked, fired from their jobs, etc. My silence in this issue is ironic given that my research and writing are often viewed as controversial and against the grain, but with this particular issue the fascist sort of quelling of any debate has given me pause from speaking out for one of the first times in my life.

Millions dealt with similar feelings as they faced an anguishing choice between their job and a medical intervention that they neither needed nor wanted—a medical intervention that would introduce unnecessary risk without commensurate benefit. Things came to a head for me in December: after twice rejecting my medical exemption, which had been signed by my physician, the University of California, Irvine, fired me for alleged noncompliance with their vaccine mandate.

Prior to covid, and even during the first year of the pandemic, I never could have imagined that the university would dismiss me and other doctors, nurses, faculty, staff, and students in this arbitrary and capricious manner. I tell my story here not because I am unique, but simply because my experience is representative of what many others—who do not necessarily have a public voice—experienced under the oppressive mandate regime. We were among early causalities of the biomedical security state, which was emerging during the pandemic.

No doctor or scientist was safe from being canceled if he or she challenged the covid regime. When our pregnant residents were worried about consulting on covid patients, the hospital administration reassured these residents that they had no elevated risks from the virus—a claim without any evidential basis at the time, and which we now know to be false. I saw the covid consults for these concerned residents, even when I was not covering the consult service.

In the early weeks of the pandemic, N95 masks were in short supply, and the hospital kept them under lock and key. Hospital administrators yelled at nurses for wearing surgical or cloth masks (this was before masks became fashionable after the CDC suggested, with little evidence, that they might help). At that early stage, nurses were doing the best they could under pressure in a situation of uncertainty. The administrators ridiculed them, not wanting to admit the real issue was that we simply did not have enough masks. I called local construction companies and sourced six hundred N95s from them. I supplied some to the residents in our department and my attending colleagues in the ER, then donated the rest to the hospital. Meanwhile the university administrators—the same ones who fired me the following year—were working safely from home and did not have to fret about PPE shortages like the frontline health care workers.

In 2020 I worked nights and weekends, uncompensated, helping the UC Office of the President draft our pandemic policies. Knowing that our ventilator triage policy was publicly sensitive, the Office of the President asked me and the chair of the committee to serve as spokespersons to answer questions about this policy and explain the principles and rationale to the public. In an ironic twist, they even provided me with media training, which came in handy later. The state of California then consulted me to improve their own ventilator triage policy after receiving public criticism for age- and disability-related discrimination issues.

I was the only faculty member at UCI who had directed courses across all four years of our medical student curriculum, and three times won the Excellence in Teaching Award from students. For many years the psychiatry clerkship I directed was the highest-rated clinical course at the medical school. I knew the medical students as well as anyone at the university. The dean asked me to address the students when they were first sent home in the early days of the pandemic.

While I strongly disagreed with the university's decision to send them home—after all, what were they here for if not to learn to practice medicine, especially during a pandemic?—I nevertheless encouraged them to continue to engage with pandemic response efforts outside the hospital. I published those remarks to encourage students at other medical schools. Our dean sent that article to the other UC medical school deans, one of whom suggested that I give the graduation speeches that year.

I'd done something similar already. In 2017, the UCI School of Medicine deans asked me to give the "White Coat Ceremony" keynote address to the incoming medical students, because, as they told me, "You are the best lecturer in the medical school." I concluded those remarks with the following advice to the incoming medical students:

> In your clinical practice, attend with particular devotion to
> the abandoned patient, the lonely patient, the patient who

suffers not only physical deprivations but human deprivations as well. In your work, always, always follow the light of your conscience, even when your decisions are unpopular. Guard against professional envy. Instead, focus your energies on serving your patients and assisting your colleagues. This will be success enough. . . .

Be absolutely convinced that you are here for a great and noble purpose. Not one of you landed here by accident. Being a physician [is] a way of life, not just a livelihood. Medicine is a *vocation*; it's not just a *career*. What is the difference, you might ask? Here's the best that I can explain it. Four years from now, when the dean hands you your medical degree, consider this: You are a physician not because you went to medical school; rather, you went to medical school because you are a physician.[71]

When I gave this speech, I was dealing with a severe chronic-pain condition from a spine injury—a condition that lasted almost five years—and could barely stand at the podium. Except when recovering from two spine surgeries, I worked every day for years at the medical center with that pain.

Everyone at the university was a fan of my work until suddenly they were not. After I challenged one of the university's covid policies, I immediately became a "threat to the health and safety of the community." No amount of empirical evidence about natural immunity or vaccine safety and efficacy mattered in the slightest. The university's leadership was not interested in scientific debate or ethical deliberation. The administration did its best to humiliate me during my period of leave and suspension. I could not even return to my office to get my belongings without being accompanied, as though I posed a safety threat simply by stepping on campus. I never had the opportunity to say goodbye to my colleagues or the students in person.

One day, I simply disappeared.[72]

• • •

As of this writing, my case challenging the university's vaccine mandate is still being litigated in the federal appellate court. From a legal perspective, the 1905 *Jacobson v. Massachusetts* Supreme Court ruling is often cited by proponents as the basis for compulsory vaccine mandates and other emergency pandemic public health measures. But *Jacobson* was a narrow ruling at the time, and the precedent it set should be construed as modest.

Justice Harlan's decision in this case over one hundred years ago upheld the states' power (not federal government's) to impose a nominal fine—$5, the equivalent of $155 today adjusted for inflation—on a person who refused to be vaccinated against smallpox during an outbreak in Boston.[73] Keep in mind that the mortality rate for smallpox at that time was 30 percent, compared to a much smaller mortality rate for covid.[74] Even though the smallpox threat was far deadlier, the state's action was clearly much less punitive and coercive than the current vaccine mandates. A $155 fine is clearly not the same as the threat of losing one's job or being excluded from attending school. But this is not the first time the *Jacobson* precedent has been misapplied by the court in acts of expansive government overreach.

The worst example was the 1927 case of *Buck v. Bell*, the notorious eugenics case mentioned in the prologue, which upheld state eugenics laws permitting involuntary sterilization. In the written ruling, Justice Holmes recast *Jacobson*'s limited holding: "The principle that sustains compulsory vaccination," he wrote, citing *Jacobson*, "is broad enough to cover cutting the Fallopian tubes." Then came the infamous line, which is worth quoting again: "Three generations of imbeciles are enough."[75] While the state laws upheld by this ruling have been legislatively reversed, this egregious Supreme Court decision has never been overturned by the court.

Our jurisprudence has evolved and developed enormously since 1905 and now includes tiered levels of scrutiny and important legal doctrines related to bodily autonomy and informed consent. Now is a good time for the Supreme Court to articulate the limits of the *Jacobson* precedent and avoid another disastrous decision like *Buck v. Bell*. Perhaps my case, or another legal challenge to vaccine mandates, will provide the court this opportunity.

Battling the CDC and the FDA

Someone once remarked that a bureaucracy is an institution that exercises enormous power over you but with no locus of responsibility. This leads to the familiar frustration, often encountered on a small scale at the local DMV, that you can go round and round in bureaucratic circles trying to troubleshoot problems or rectify unfair practices. No actual person seems to be able to help you get to the bottom of things—even if a well-meaning employee sincerely wants to assist you. With the advent of vaccine mandates for competent adults in 2021, the world turned into one enormous bureaucracy—like being stuck inside a global DMV.

"The ideal bureaucrat is identical to a computer," Mattias Desmet wrote. "They strictly adhere to the logic of their system without being 'distracted' by the individuality of the people they 'assist.'" This is why, he explains, the bureaucratic system generates the same kinds of frustrations as a computer: "We are confronted with a mechanical Other who is in no way sensitive to our individuality as human beings. A computer is not so much an unfair or unjust Other; it is an Other who imposes a relentless logic." Desmet points out that, in this respect, the computer and the bureaucratic functionary resemble the ideal totalitarian leader, who "strictly and ruthlessly imposes his logic on the population."[76]

Here's how the bureaucratic dynamic played out with vaccine mandates. Dissecting the anatomy of coercion, in which totalizing power was exerted with no locus of responsibility, we discover the following closed-loop system—relentless in its "logic" and unfeeling in its application to individuals. The CDC made vaccine recommendations. But the ethically crucial distinction between a recommendation and a mandate immediately collapsed when institutions (for example, a government agency, business, employer, university, or school) required employees or contractors to be vaccinated, based on the CDC recommendation.

If one tried, as I did, to contest the rationality of these mandates, for example, in federal court, the mandating institution just pointed back to CDC recommendation as the rational basis for their mandate. The courts typically agreed, deferring to the CDC's authority on public health. The city, school, business, and so forth thus disclaimed all responsibility for the mandate decision: *We're just following CDC recommendations, after all. What can we do?* But moving up the food chain, the CDC likewise disclaimed responsibility: *We don't make policy; we just make recommendations.*

Meanwhile, the vaccine manufacturer was immune and indemnified from all liability under federal law—specifically the 2005 PREP Act and the 1986 National Childhood Vaccine Injury Act. It's no use going to them if their product—a product that you did not freely decide to take—harms you. By this time those of us trying to question mandates were dizzy from going round in circles trying to identify the actual decision-maker. It was impossible to pinpoint the relevant authority. We knew and felt that enormous power was being exercised over our bodies and our health, but with no locus of responsibility for the decision and no liability for the outcomes. Millions were then left to contend with the consequences of a decision that nobody claims to have made. The only certainty is that *we* did not make the decision and we were never given the choice.

Following this pattern, the university's only legal defense in my case was that the CDC had not yet acknowledged natural immunity for covid. The issue of natural immunity is a helpful lens through which to understand the CDC's profound institutional failures during the pandemic. It required some digging to find out why our leading public health agency was ignoring such a basic scientific fact and instead taking a flat-earth approach to covid policy. The science on the efficacy and durability of natural immunity was very strong by the time I filed my suit and only became more compelling with each passing month as my case dragged on in the courts. Yet the CDC continued to recommend vaccination for those who had already had covid. Vaccine mandates across the country likewise ignored natural immunity, mostly because the CDC was ignoring it. The reasons are rooted in some of the central features of the biomedical security state.

There were several political reasons the CDC continued to ignore the scientific evidence on this issue. First, public health officials worried that acknowledging natural immunity would lead people to deliberately try to get infected with the virus instead of getting vaccinated. But of course, the question was not about whether people should try to acquire natural immunity by intentionally getting infected; nobody was suggesting this. It was about the level of immunity afforded to those who had already recovered from covid. Consistent with the propaganda-based approach to public messaging, informational accuracy was sacrificed in the interest of forcing predetermined behavioral outcomes.

Second, public health officials worried that establishing whether or not a potential vaccine recipient has already had covid was too inefficient and cumbersome. Officials rejected anything that might slow the efficiency of vaccination campaigns or complicate the simplistic "needle in every arm" public message. But they could simply have placed the burden of proof on the vaccine recipients to show proof of prior infection. Some people with prior infection may still want the vaccine while others may choose to forego it. We could have easily provided the option of presenting previous screening results, medical records, or results from antibody testing or a T cell test (which remains positive after antibodies inevitably decline). This one-size-fits-all approach to public health, where strict controls apply indiscriminately to entire populations, is also characteristic of the biomedical security state.

Third—and this was the part not said out loud—public health officials worried that acknowledging natural immunity would amount to admitting the failure of their policies, which were implemented to prevent people from getting infected. The two most basic numbers in immunology are incidence and prevalence: the former designates the rate of *new* cases over time, whereas the latter designates the rate of *total* cases over time. Once the CDC acknowledges natural immunity, the obvious question is then about prevalence: How many Americans had already been infected with covid since the pandemic began?

That more than two years into the pandemic we still did not have a clear answer to this most basic question was astonishing. It could easily have been answered by randomly sampled, population-based, T cell testing or antibody testing sampled sequentially in population-based cohorts every few months. This was basic epidemiology the CDC should have been conducting throughout the pandemic. If our public health authorities got back to epidemiological basics and did these studies, most epidemiologists estimated that by the end of the omicron wave, somewhere between 65 percent and 75 percent of the population had natural immunity, including many who were vaccinated (which, as it happens, artificially elevated estimates of vaccine efficacy).

For public health officials who would never admit that they were wrong, this would be clear evidence of their failed policies. Despite draconian lockdowns, social distancing, masking, scrubbing of surfaces, plastic barriers, and so on, the virus nevertheless still did what respiratory viruses do: most Americans got infected anyways. Self-interested public health agencies would have seen this as bad news, rather than celebrating it as progress toward herd immunity. This admission would have undermined the entire biosecurity approach to pandemic management that the CDC had embraced.

In April 2022 the CDC finally published a seroprevalence study of anti-nucleocapsid antibodies, which are produced in response to infection but not in response to covid vaccines. They found that at least 75 percent of children had already been infected with covid, as had at least 64 percent of adults under age fifty.[77] The silver lining was that, of the huge number of people who had been infected with covid, 99.8 percent had survived, including 99.9996 percent of those under age fifty.[78] Professor

John Ioannidis of Stanford demonstrated early on that the infection fatality rate of covid by age bracket was extremely low for healthy children and adults under age seventy.[79] This information alone was sufficient to demonstrate that lockdowns, vaccine mandates, and vaccine passports should never have been considered in the first place. That these measures were almost universally adopted suggests that this decision had little to do with public health.

There were other political and financial considerations unduly influencing public agencies like the CDC on covid policies. Most obvious was the fact that acknowledging natural immunity would cut the profits of a $100 billion covid vaccine industry by more than half. I quipped at the time that they would recognize natural immunity when someone figured out how to monetize it. Of course, these factors should not have influenced the CDC; but as we will see when we examine regulatory capture later in this chapter, our three-letter federal agencies are unduly influenced by the pharmaceutical companies they are supposed to regulate. Conflicts of interest abound.

Against these nonscientific roadblocks, which have little to do with public health and sound policymaking, in 2021 I began exploring how responsible scientists could help move the needle on the CDC's position. Attempts to do so had so far met with stonewalling. The CDC's preferred response to challenges from scientists was stony silence. I coordinated a group of academic physicians and scientists to take legal action against the CDC, petitioning the agency to acknowledge natural immunity.

In May of that year, the CDC had changed its recommendations to loosen restrictions on fully vaccinated individuals, but the recommendations did not acknowledge those with infection-induced immunity. My lawyer on the UCI case, Aaron Siri, submitted a letter—with a detailed declaration by my colleague Peter McCullough—detailing the robust scientific evidence for natural immunity and demanding that the CDC include covid-recovered individuals in the same category as the vaccinated.

In response, the CDC sent a dismissive two-sentence form letter that addressed none of the scientific issues raised in the petitioners' letter. The

CDC thanked Siri for his "interest in 2019 Coronavirus Disease" and provided a link to the same policy that Siri had extensively critiqued in his letter. The upside of this nonresponsive response, however, was that it allowed Siri to formally petition the CDC, which he did with a letter on July 6. As it happens, only two types of people can take legal action in federal court against the CDC: the agency's own employees or a lawyer who has received an official response from the CDC to a specific type of petition, which was the case here.

The CDC did not bother to respond to our July 6 follow-up letter, even though they were required by law to do so. Siri's team sent another letter on September 15 delicately pointing this out and attaching a helpful bibliography of fifty-six additional studies published on natural immunity since the original letter—studies that only further confirmed our initial case. The CDC finally responded on September 17, denying the petition.

This denial was based on one engineered study looking at infection rates in Kentucky, which the CDC had just published. The timing suggested the study was ginned up in reaction to our petition. The Kentucky study did not, however, examine the relevant comparison groups: vaccinated versus covid-recovered. Instead, all the subjects examined in the study were covid-recovered and half of these were subsequently vaccinated. Siri's next letter included a thorough critique and contextualization of this irrelevant study—a transparently engineered bit of research that was so methodologically embarrassing that even vaccine proponents no longer bothered to cite it. Siri also pointed out that the CDC's response made no mention of the more than fifty other relevant studies that petitioners had summarized and submitted to the CDC for review.

What came next was interesting. Siri's team—with help from several academic physicians and scientists I coordinated from UCLA, UCSF, Brown, Stanford, and other institutes—submitted a reply on October 21. The letter pointed out that the agency's failure to recognize natural immunity was causing an incredible level of reputational harm to the CDC and undermining public trust in all CDC recommendations. The letter concluded by indicating that we, the petitioners, were prepared to take legal action in federal court if the CDC continued to fail to act on our petition. As of this writing, our team is waiting on additional information regarding the CDC's flawed Kentucky study, with pending Freedom of Information Act petitions for relevant documents, before our next legal steps.

Of note, one of our FOIA requests to the CDC was for the following information: "Documents reflecting any documented case of an individual who: (1) never received a COVID-19 vaccine; (2) was infected with COVID-19 once, recovered, and then later became infected again; and (3) transmitted SARS-CoV-2 to another person when reinfected." The CDC's response was telling: "A search of our records failed to reveal any documents pertaining to your request. The CDC Emergency Operations Center (EOC) conveyed that this information is not collected."

This suggested not only that the agency's policy recommendation for vaccinating individuals with natural immunity (on the presumption that they need vaccination to protect others) lacked the tiniest shred of data to support it, but it also revealed that the CDC showed no interest in even attempting to collect such data. Nevertheless, all the vaccine mandates that ignore natural immunity, including the UC mandate, relied on this CDC recommendation as their foundation. Thousands like me lost our jobs over this issue, and round and round in circles we go looking for any shred of scientific justification.

● ● ●

I also crossed swords with the FDA in 2021. According to the World Health Organization (WHO), "out of 86 clinical trials for 20 COVID-19 vaccines, 12% of clinical trial protocols were made publically available."[80] In September 2021 I organized thirty academic physicians and scientists to form Public Health and Medical Professionals for Transparency. This group included, among other luminaries, Harvey Risch of Yale, Andrew Bostom of Brown, Joseph Ladapo of UCLA (now Surgeon

General of Florida), Paul Alexander, formerly of HHS and WHO, Aditi Bhargava of UCSF, and other scientists from the United States, Canada, Denmark, Australia, Germany, and the University of Oxford in the United Kingdom.

We submitted a Freedom of Information Act (FOIA) request to the FDA for all the clinical trials data relied upon to authorize Pfizer's covid vaccine. This information was not available while the vaccine was only approved under emergency use authorization (EUA). But under federal law, the FDA was required to make this data publicly available once the vaccine, Comirnaty, received approval, which happened in August that year. The law is crystal clear on this point: our FOIA request was not legally complicated, and the FDA's lawyers at the Department of Justice were aware of this.

As our website describes: "The organization takes no position on the data other than that it should be made publicly available to allow independent experts to conduct their own review and analyses. Any data received will be made public."[81] We have made good on this promise. Our FOIA request should have been uncontroversial since transparency is widely regarded as a core ethical principle of all public health initiatives. It is one of the central ethical principles articulated, for example, in the University of California's "Allocation of Scarce Critical Resources under Crisis Standards of Care," the ventilator triage policy that I helped draft for the UC hospitals in 2020.[82]

In response the FDA indicated it would release five hundred pages per month. Doing the math, this meant it would take seventy-five years to release the data the FDA reviewed in only 108 days. The federal judge rejected the FDA's absurd timeline and ordered the agency to release the data within eight months. In his order, the judge wrote eloquently on the central role of transparency from government agencies in a functioning democracy:

"Open government is fundamentally an American issue"—it is neither a Republican nor a Democrat issue. As James Madison wrote, "[a] popular Government, without popular information, or the means of acquiring it, is but a Prologue to a Farce or a Tragedy; or, perhaps, both. Knowledge will forever govern ignorance: And a people who mean to be their own Governors, must arm themselves with the power which knowledge gives."[83]

After the judge ordered the FDA to release the data, Pfizer got worried and attempted to intervene. The company requested permission to redact the documents prior to their release. That Pfizer would make this request was not surprising; what was shocking, however, was that the Department of Justice lawyers representing the FDA concurred with Pfizer, petitioning the court to allow the company to assist with redactions. The judge declined this absurd request.

As of this writing, we continue to get additional documents each month, and researchers are working through hundreds of thousands of pages. The released documents included, among other relevant pieces of previously undisclosed information, data on adverse reactions reported in the first three months of the mass vaccination campaign. That document noted, "Due to the large numbers of spontaneous adverse event reports received for the product [the covid vaccine]," Pfizer was prioritizing documentation of the most "serious cases." To handle the high number of adverse event reports, "Pfizer has onboarded approximately 600 additional full-time employees (FTEs). More are joining each month with an expected total of more than 1800 additional FTE resources by the end of June 2021." The numbers showed: "Cumulatively, through 28 February 2021, there was a total of 42,086 case reports (25,379 medically confirmed and 16,707 non-medically confirmed) containing 158,893 [adverse] events." Also of concern, data released revealed that out of thirty-two pregnancies with a known outcome following vaccination, twenty-eight resulted in fetal death.[84]

Given that reporting was voluntary, cumbersome, and time-consuming for busy clinicians, the adverse events listed were surely underreported; but the numbers were nevertheless alarming. Vaccine adverse events included many organ systems beyond the cardiac problems that have so far received attention: "Nervous system disorders (25,957), Musculoskeletal and connective tissue disorders (17,283), Gastrointestinal disorders (14,096), Skin and subcutaneous tissue disorders (8,476), Respiratory, thoracic and mediastinal disorders (8,848), Infections and infestations (4,610), Injury, poisoning and procedural complications (5,590), and Investigations (3,693)." An appendix listing the various types of reported adverse reactions consisted of nine solid pages of text describing countless medically serious conditions.[85] I have never seen anything like it anywhere in the medical literature.

For any other product, the FDA would have immediately halted its use.

The Pfizer data demonstrate that risks were known that were not disclosed to recipients during the mass vaccination campaign. Pfizer and the FDA knew about these adverse events, which are dose-dependent, that is, they worsen with subsequent boosters. They also knew that all-cause mortality was higher in the vaccine group than the placebo group, and they knew that this mortality among the vaccinated was associated with cardiotoxicity. They knew that these vaccines would not protect us against infection, viral replication, or transmission. They knew the vaccine was tested neither in pregnant women nor in older populations that are at highest risk from covid. They knew that their efficacy claims were overstated.

Their lack of transparency and disclosure of these risks not only undermined informed consent, which requires accurate disclosure of relevant information, but may indeed legally constitute fraud. Vaccine manufacturers' immunity from liability does not shield the company in the case of fraud—deliberate withholding of relevant known information—so this may be one way to pierce the indemnity veil and hold the corporation accountable for damages.

That scientists and physicians such as the group I coordinated must take our three-letter agencies like the CDC and FDA to court to get them to acknowledge basic scientific facts or share their data is a sign of the advanced decay of these agencies. I will close this chapter with a brief account of the mechanisms of institutional capture and corruption that now afflict the CDC, FDA, and NIH—all divisions of the federal Department of Health and Human Services (HHS). In the wake of the pandemic, it's clear that these agencies no longer work for the taxpayers that fund them. The question then arises, whose interests are they serving?

Regulatory Capture

Pharmaceutical companies now exercise outsized influence over media and government agencies. Pharma, it turns out, pays for the science we are told to trust. To begin, we need to appreciate the sheer size of pharmaceutical companies: "These days, Pfizer rakes in $81 billion a year, making it the 28th most valuable company in the world. Johnson & Johnson ranks 15th, with $93.77 billion. To put things into perspective, that makes said companies wealthier than most countries in the world," allowing them to spend more on lobbying than any other industry. The covid vaccines alone have generated $100 billion in profits. "In 2020, more than two-thirds of Congress—72 senators and 302 House of Representatives members—cashed a campaign check from a pharma company," journalist Rebecca Strong reported.[86]

In response to a FOIA request from a government watchdog group, it recently came to light that the federal government paid $1 billion in taxpayer dollars to hundreds of media companies to advertise the covid vaccines. As you might expect, those same outlets provided uniformly positive coverage of the vaccines and downplayed concerns about safety and efficacy. Recipients of government advertising dollars that benefitted pharma included the *New York Post*, *Los Angeles Times*, and *Washington Post*; ABC, CBS, CNN, Fox News, MSNBC, and NBC; BuzzFeed, Newsmax, and hundreds of local newspapers and television stations. Commercials funded by the Department of Health and Human Services featured celebrities like singer Elton John and actor Michael Caine.[87]

The government used taxpayer dollars to: (1) fund the development of covid vaccines, (2) test covid vaccines, (3) approve these vaccines, (4) distribute these vaccines, (5) guarantee markets for covid vaccines through mandates, (6) incentivize vaccine uptake via lotteries and other giveaways, and (7) advertise these vaccines. Vaccine manufacturers were immune from all liability for any harms caused by their products, thanks to federal law. Not a bad business model for Pfizer and Moderna. But where is the return on investment for the taxpayers? We were rewarded with vaccines that did not stop infection or transmission of the virus and whose efficacy against disease waned rapidly. And many were rewarded with serious side effects—including death—for which there is no compensation.

The federal feeding trough of advertising revenue to media conglomerates was mere gravy on top of the pharmaceutical advertising dollars flowing to these media companies. Prior to 1985 direct-to-consumer advertising of prescription drugs was prohibited by federal law. Pharma could market their drugs to prescribing physicians in medical journals but could not advertise directly to patients. After all, these were prescription medications—not cosmetics, shoes, fast food, or soda.

The FDA relaxed regulations again in 1997 to permit broadcast drug advertisements, after which we began to see "ask your doctor about Viagra" commercials routinely. The United States and New Zealand remain the only countries where prescription pharmaceutical television ads are legal. The rest of the world rightly finds these ads shockingly bizarre. Following the change in 1997, pharma became the largest advertiser for all major media organizations.[88] This buys considerable influence in the newsroom—whether media companies acknowledge this or not.

Most biomedical research is paid for by pharmaceutical companies. The *New England Journal of Medicine* found that 82 percent of their seventy-three published studies of new drugs in one year had been funded by the pharmaceutical company selling the drug. More than two-thirds of studies had authors who were employees of the respective pharmaceutical company, and half of the studies had lead researchers who accepted money from a drug company. Furthermore, a 2017 report in the *British Medical Journal* showed that about half of medical-journal editors receive payments from drug companies, with the average payment around $28,000. The investigation found 80 percent of study authors failed to disclose pharma payments totaling millions of dollars.[89]

The revolving door, where FDA officials land handsome gigs at the companies they formerly regulated, is well-documented. A 2018 report in *Science* found that more than two-thirds of FDA reviewers later ended up at the same companies they had been reviewing products for while working for government.[90] Similarly, a study published in the *British Medical Journal* by my colleague Vinay Prasad of UCSF revealed that from 2001 to 2010, almost two-thirds of reviewers who left the FDA later worked or consulted for the pharmaceutical industry.[91] During that nine-year period, over one-quarter of all the FDA reviewers left their federal oversight posts to work for the industry they only recently regulated. Moreover, "nine out of 10 of its past commissioners between 2006 and 2019 went on to secure roles linked with pharmaceutical companies, and its 11th and most recent, Stephen Hahn, is working for Flagship Pioneering, a company that acts as an incubator for new biopharmaceutical companies."[92]

The revolving door creates a small coterie of mutual backscratchers moving seamlessly from government to industry and back—a form of public-private cronyism. This is one of the mechanisms by which pharmaceutical companies capture the agencies that are supposed ensure that the corporate profit motive does not trump the public good. As we will see in the next chapter, these kinds of "public-private partnerships"—a euphemism for corporatism—are a central feature of the biomedical security state.

The NIH likewise maintains strong industry ties that create serious conflicts of interest. In 2018 it was revealed that a $100 million NIH study on the benefits of moderate drinking was funded by the beer and liquor industry.[93] Closer to our own day, most people are still unaware that the NIAID, Fauci's division of the NIH, owns half the patent on the Moderna vaccine, among thousands of other pharma patents.[94] Rather than providing grants to university-based investigators to run the clinical trials on their own Moderna vaccine, the NIH conducted this research internally, a clear conflict of interest. The NIAID will earn millions from this vaccine's revenue, with several NIH employees (and their heirs) personally receiving up to $150,000 annually from Moderna vaccine sales.[95]

In May 2022 documents obtained by a FOIA request from Open the Books, a nonprofit organization dedicated to investigating and disclosing government expenditures, revealed that NIH director Francis Collins, NIAID director Anthony Fauci, and Fauci's deputy director, Clifford Lane, all received royalties from pharmaceutical companies between 2009 and 2014. Open the Books estimates that "between fiscal years 2010 and 2020, more than $350 million in royalties were paid by third-parties to the agency and NIH scientists—who are credited as co-inventors."

A plausible argument can be made for this practice; however, in the years they received payments, Collins, Fauci, and Lane were administrators, not researchers, at the NIH, with no plausible claim to be scientific codiscoverers. The exact amount they earned from royalties was redacted from the released documents.[96] Even after citizens take legal action, the NIH steadfastly refuses to maintain public transparency.

There was a time not so long ago when the CDC could not take money from the pharmaceutical industry. But in 1992 the agency discovered a loophole in federal law that allowed them to accept pharma contributions through a nonprofit called the CDC Foundation. The money started flowing immediately: from 2014 through 2018, the CDC Foundation received $79.6 million from pharmaceutical corporations like Pfizer, Biogen, and Merck. Likewise, the NIH Foundation allows private money to flow to this public institution, introducing undue influence over research funding.[97]

The NIH funds research, the CDC makes public health recommendations, but the FDA is the ultimate gatekeeper as the agency that approves new drugs or vaccines before they go to market. The real payoff therefore comes when pharma cozies up to the FDA. As with the CDC, there was a time when the FDA could not accept pharma dollars. That changed in 1992 when Congress altered the FDA's funding mechanisms to allow for pharmaceutical companies to pay "user fees" to speed up the approval process for their products. The following year, in 1993, pharma fees paid for 27 percent of the FDA's scientific review budgets. By 2017 pharma paid for 75 percent of this budget.[98]

Rebecca Strong explained how other backdoor bribes slip easily through the cracks at the FDA:

> A 2018 *Science* investigation found that 40 out of 107 physician advisors on the FDA's committees received more than $10,000 from big pharma companies trying to get their drugs approved, with some banking up to $1 million or more. The FDA claims it has a well-functioning system to identify and prevent these possible conflicts of interest. Unfortunately, their system only works for spotting payments *before* advisory panels meet, and the *Science* investigation showed many FDA panel members get their payments after the fact.[99]

It would be beyond naïve to believe this routine flow of pharma money fails to influence our federal three-letter agencies—the NIH, CDC, and FDA—the very agencies responsible to citizens for our public health and for regulating the pharmaceutical industry. I will return in the final chapter to this issue of regulatory capture when discussing potential policy solutions to this serious problem.

Unfortunately, the situation is no better at the international level. For most of its history since its founding in 1948, the WHO could accept donations only from member states. In 2005 they changed their policies to permit private funding. Today only 20 percent of its funding comes from member states, with 80 percent coming from private sources, including pharmaceutical companies. Thirteen percent of the WHO's funding ($300 million annually) comes from the Bill & Melinda Gates Foundation—a larger contribution than that of the United States government during the first year of the pandemic.[100]

Lawrence Gostin, director of WHO's Collaborating Center on National and Global Health Law, expressed concerns to a reporter in 2020 regarding these funding arrangements: "By [Gates] wielding such influence, it could steer WHO priorities." Gostin also pointed out that this "would enable a single rich philanthropist to set the global health agenda." At the WHO's founding as an intergovernmental organization, such a situation "would have been unimaginable," he said.[101] The WHO's list of donors also includes AstraZeneca, Bayer, Pfizer, Johnson & Johnson, and Merck.[102]

● ● ●

This backdrop is helpful to contextualize the data integrity and patient-safety problems with Pfizer's covid vaccine clinical trial revealed in the *British Medical Journal* in 2021. The courageous whistleblower Brook Jackson, regional director of Ventavia, a private company that conducted the clinical trial for Pfizer, allowed us to peek behind the curtain. Jackson alleged that "the company falsified data, unblinded patients, employed inadequately trained vaccinators, and was slow to follow up on adverse events reported in Pfizer's pivotal phase III trial." Jackson also witnessed unreported or incorrectly reported vaccine adverse events, protocol deviations, informed consent problems, and mislabeling of lab specimens.[103] Jackson told Rebecca Strong in an interview, "When missing data points were discovered the information was fabricated, including forged signatures on the informed consent forms."

Jackson "filed a complaint with the FDA" on September 25, 2020. Ventavia fired her "a few hours later" saying she was "not a good fit." (This pattern is starting to sound familiar.) The FDA never investigated her complaint and instead gave the vaccine emergency use authorization a little over two months later. Ventavia, by the way, also "handled the clinical trials for the Moderna, Johnson & Johnson, and Novavax" covid vaccines.[104]

The *New England Journal of Medicine* published the positive phase 3 study on Pfizer's vaccine, the basis for the FDA's emergency use authorization of this product.[105] Rebecca Strong investigated the study authors' conflicts of interests and found that "of the 29 authors, 18 are employees of Pfizer and hold stock in the company, one received a research grant from Pfizer during the study, and two reported being paid 'personal fees' by Pfizer." She also noted, "In another 2021 study on the Pfizer vaccine, seven of the 15 authors are employees of and hold stock in Pfizer. The other eight authors received financial support from Pfizer during the study."[106] The pivotal *New England Journal of Medicine* article provided only a small slice of the data collected in the clinical trial. As recounted in the previous section, my colleagues and I had to battle in court to get the rest of the Pfizer study data from the FDA.

Having read the *British Medical Journal* story about Brook Jackson's whistleblower case and spoken to her on a couple of occasions, I was not entirely shocked when another whistleblower from Argentina reached out to me later in 2021 with a strikingly similar story. Augusto Roux, a previously fit-and-healthy thirty-six-year-old lawyer who worked in the supreme court of Argentina, was a participant in Pfizer's vaccine clinical trial in his home country. Roux had volunteered for the study to protect his mother who suffered from emphysema. Due in large part to its lax regulatory system and a political culture of bribery, Argentina hosts many clinical trials for Big Pharma. The story Roux recounted to me of his experience echoed Jackson's account of mismanagement and malfeasance. In his case, however, he was not an employee but a research subject who was medically harmed during the trial—harm that the company then attempted to cover up.

Dr. David Healy subsequently published an extensive and medically detailed account of Roux's vaccine injury in the clinical trial, the company's cover-up, and the falsification of his data.[107] The senior doctor in the hospital where Roux was admitted for treatment diagnosed him with a vaccine injury (pericarditis), confirmed by all the requisite testing and clearly documented in his medical record. Despite this the research investigators falsified his diagnosis in the study data, incorrectly recording his adverse event as anxiety. In addition the lead clinical investigator, Fernando Polack, a pediatrician with no training in psychiatric diagnosis, "had the mental health misdiagnosis added to Roux's actual medical records." This information surfaced because Roux, a lawyer, sued to get his clinical trials records and his medical records, initiating a process that last over a year.[108] One commentator noted:

> Recall that Polack was the first author on the December, 2020 NEJM paper on the safety and efficacy of the vaccine. He is also one of the directors of i-trials, the site management organization paid handsomely by Pfizer to run the trial in Argentina (the largest site of the trial by far). If he raised an alarm about the vaccine safety, his company would have lost a ton of money and would be an unlikely choice by any company to run any trials in the future. So to say that he had an interest in achieving a positive trial outcome would be quite an understatement.[109]

The study researchers also misdiagnosed Roux as having covid within a week of vaccination, despite zero laboratory, clinical, or radiological evidence of infection.[110] Coding him as infected with covid a week after vaccination meant that the study did not have to count him as a covid case in the vaccinated, because the study defined fully vaccinated as fourteen days after the second dose. As far as the trial was concerned, after they misidentified him as a covid case, his entire case simply—and conveniently—disappeared from the data. Roux told me he observed other trial participants who suffered the same fate.

Along with Roux, 302 trial participants from the vaccine arm (including over 200 from Buenos Aires, the largest site) and 52 from the placebo arm dropped out of the study and were not counted in the data. As Dr. Healy noted, "Someone like Eric Rubin, the editor-in-chief of

NEJM [*New England Journal of Medicine*], or a senior honcho in FDA, you'd imagine should ideally get the contact details of these 302 who have disappeared and get their side of the story. Roux and a few hundred others are the real raw data."[111]

Roux wrote to the FDA and its European counterpart, the EMA, in late 2020 explaining what had happened to him and seeking redress. His pleas were entirely ignored. He also filed a VAERS report in November 2020 and received a confirmation with a temporary VAERS number. However, his report seems not to have made it into the VAERS system.

Recall that while pharmaceutical companies are liable for the harms caused by their medications, under the federal Public Readiness and Emergency Preparedness (PREP) Act they enjoy near-total immunity from liability for their vaccines. In the case of covid vaccines, victims of vaccine injuries also cannot be compensated through the National Vaccine Injury Compensation Program, which was set up to offer vaccine injury payouts (in exchange for signing a nondisclosure agreement to never mention your vaccine injury) after the federal government indemnified pharmaceutical companies for these injuries in 1987. If you have been harmed by a covid vaccine you can seek legal redress neither from the NIH that studied it, nor from the FDA that authorized it, nor from the CDC that recommended it, nor from the company or agency that mandated it, nor from company that produced it.

Like Augusto Roux, you have no recourse. You don't count. You simply disappear.

CHAPTER 3

Locked In: The Coming Technocratic Dystopia

The nightmare of the brave new world need not fear old-fashioned torture and gas chambers. The universal totalitarian institution will be the hospital, and the universal uniform of the new elites will be the white physician-therapist coat. The brave new world will be . . . one vast hospital.

—*Philip Rieff,* The Crisis of the Officer Class

Prior to and during the pandemic, climate change was reframed from an environmental issue to a public health issue. Soon it may be declared a public health crisis. Imagine a few years hence you receive a text on your phone: this notification explains that your carbon footprint is 23 percent above others' in your age/race/gender category for your geographic region. The message informs you that you have eighteen months to transition to an electric vehicle; otherwise you will be taxed an additional $0.90 per gallon of gas.

While that gas tax is steep, you default to that "option" because you simply cannot afford an electric vehicle. Six months later, you receive another notification that your individualized carbon footprint tax will double to $1.80 per gallon if you don't convert over, which hurts your wallet even more but does not change your financial prospects for a new electric car. A year later, an algorithm in the cloud decides that since you have still not converted to an electric vehicle, you now cannot buy gas.

After all, each of us is responsible for population health and safety. "We're all in this together."

The biomedical security state will soon have the necessary infrastructure in place to implement policies of this kind, including, as we will explore in this chapter, digital IDs and central bank digital currencies. These will be tied to digital health-passport systems already tested and deployed during the pandemic. While the technology for this is already available, a skeptic might still ask, are we really in danger of heading toward an increasingly authoritarian technocracy? Are we likely to live in a society that would deploy these biomedical surveillance tools in this manner? In this chapter, we will explore these and other questions about the near future. The epilogue will paint a picture of where the biomedical security state will lead in the next eight years if it continues to advance unopposed.

Since 1975 a Swedish nonprofit called the International Institute for Democracy and Electoral Assistance (IDEA) has been carefully tracking metrics to measure authoritarian global trends. According to its analysis, in the last few years the number of countries that are becoming more authoritarian is three times the number of countries moving in the other direction toward open democracies. The year 2021 was the fifth in a row that saw overall authoritarian gains, the longest continuous period trending in that direction since IDEA began tracking these metrics almost fifty years ago. IDEA warned in its annual *Global State of Democracy Report 2021*: "The world is becoming more authoritarian as nondemocratic regimes become even more brazen in their repression and many democratic governments suffer from backsliding by adopting their tactics of restricting free speech and weakening the rule of law, exacerbated by what threatens to become a 'new normal' of COVID-19 restrictions."[1]

In his classic dystopian novel *Ninetee Eighty-Four*, George Orwell famously wrote, "If you want a picture of the future, imagine a boot stamping on a human face—for ever."[2] This striking image served as a potent symbol for totalitarianism in the twentieth century. But with the advent of digital health passports in the emerging biomedical security state, the new symbol of totalitarian repression is "not a boot, but an algorithm in the cloud: emotionless, impervious to appeal, silently shaping the biomass," as Caylan Ford recently observed.[3] In our technocratic society, the new digital surveillance and control mechanisms will be no less oppressive for being virtual rather than physical.

Consider the following trends during the pandemic. Contact-tracing apps proliferated, with at least 120 different location-tracking apps used in seventy-one different states, and sixty other digital contact-tracing measures used in thirty-eight countries. We still lack any evidence that contact-tracing apps or other methods of digital surveillance helped to slow the spread of covid. But as with so many of our pandemic policies, the absence of evidence to support them did not deter their widespread use.[4]

Other advanced technologies were deployed to enable what one commentator called, with a nod to Orwell's boot, "the stomp reflex": a phrase that designates governments' propensity to abuse emergency powers. Twenty-two countries used surveillance drones to monitor their populations for covid rule-breakers; twenty-eight countries used internet censorship; thirteen countries resorted to internet shutdowns to manage populations during the pandemic. Several countries besides China deployed facial-recognition technologies to track down dissenters. Thirty-two countries deployed militaries or military ordnances to enforce rules, actions which included casualties. In Angola, for example, police shot and killed several citizens while imposing a lockdown.[5] All for the sake of their health, of course.

The United Kingdom's National Health Service (NHS) took data mining of private health information to the next level by attempting to monetize it. Strapped for cash, the NHS recently planned to digitize and sell the private health data of all fifty-five million users to private companies and third parties. People were technically allowed to opt out; however, the public was informed only shortly before the opt-out period expired, leaving citizens little time to act. The whole scheme was abandoned only after the *Financial Times* ran an exposé in May 2021.[6]

Although the NHS never fully cashed in on the sale of citizens' private health data, by the time the plan was shelved the NHS had already shared data with dozens of companies around the world. This included unauthorized sharing of data of over 80 percent of the patients who had specifically elected to opt out.[7] Oops.

A few months later *The Guardian* revealed that the NHS was sharing facial recognition data, collected from the NHS App's vaccine certificate, with law enforcement agencies and undisclosed companies. One expert in surveillance law, who asked not to be named, told *The Guardian* that such information was desirable to United Kingdom and foreign intelligence services, and if it proved useful they would likely share it with the U.S. National Security Agency. The director of the nonprofit firm Foxglove, a team of lawyers that investigates harmful uses of technology, commented, "We should all also reflect on whether we're heading towards a world where people have to use their faces just to walk into the supermarket or the pharmacy or the nightclub."[8]

Biosecurity Newspeak

George Orwell explored the power of language to shape our thinking, including the power of intentionally sloppy language to distort thought. He articulated these concerns not only in his novels *Animal Farm* and *Nineteen Eighty-Four* but also in his classic essay "Politics and the English Language," where he argues that "if thought corrupts language, language can also corrupt thought."[9]

The totalitarian regime depicted in *Nineteen Eighty-Four*, the Party, requires citizens to communicate in Newspeak, a carefully controlled language of simplified grammar and restricted vocabulary. This language is designed to limit the individual's ability to think and articulate subversive concepts such as personal identity, self-expression, and free will. With Newspeak's bastardization of English, complete thoughts are reduced to dumbed-down terms conveying only simplistic meaning. Newspeak purposefully eliminates the possibility of nuance: it renders impossible the consideration and communication of subtlety or shades of meaning. The Party also intends with Newspeak's short words to make speech hypnotic, physically automatic, and largely unconscious, which further erodes the potential for critical thought.

The novel's character Syme discusses his editorial work on the latest edition of the Newspeak Dictionary:

> By 2050—earlier, probably—all real knowledge of Old-speak [standard English] will have disappeared. The whole literature of the past will have been destroyed. Chaucer, Shakespeare, Milton, Byron—they'll exist only in Newspeak versions, not merely changed into something different, but actually contradictory of what they used to be. Even the literature of The Party will change. Even the slogans will change. How could you have a slogan like Freedom is Slavery when the concept of freedom has been abolished? The whole climate of thought will be different. In fact, there will be no thought, as we understand it now. Orthodoxy means not thinking—not needing to think. Orthodoxy is unconsciousness.[10]

Newspeak includes many simplified word contractions: *joycamp* is a labor camp; *Miniluv* is the Ministry of Love, where secret police torture and interrogate dissidents; *Minipax* is the Ministry of Peace, responsible for waging war; *oldthink* refers to ideas from the time before the Party's revolution, such as objectivity and rationality; *pornosec* is the pornography production section of the Ministry of Truth's fiction department; *thinkpol* is the Thought Police, the secret police force of the Party; and *unperson* refers to someone who has been executed, whose very existence is subsequently erased from history and memory. Kind of like canceled.

The novel's protagonist, Winston Smith, eventually learns the function of these terms and the purpose of their manifest contradictions:

Even the names of the four Ministries by which we are governed exhibit a sort of impudence in their deliberate reversal
of the facts. The Ministry of Peace concerns itself with war,
the Ministry of Truth with lies, the Ministry of Love with
torture and the Ministry of Plenty with starvation. These
contradictions are not accidental, nor do they result from
ordinary hypocrisy; they are deliberate exercises in double-
think. For it is only by reconciling contradictions that power
can be retained indefinitely.[11]

Smith, who works at the Ministry of Truth, eventually realizes that
the function of overt propaganda, with its banal and repetitious slogans,
is precisely to confuse and humiliate people. Smith's job is to drop inconvenient documents (like last week's newspaper) down an incinerator
called the Memory Hole, so that the information contained therein can
be promptly erased and forgotten. Last week, the newspaper proclaimed
that Eurasia is Oceania's ally. But that went down the Memory Hole:
today's newspaper proclaims that Oceania is at war with Eurasia. What
is more, Oceania *has always* been at war with Eurasia.[12]

One month we are told that vaccines stop viral transmission. The
next month we are told by the same talking heads that vaccines do not
stop viral transmission. What is more, these vaccines were never meant
to stop viral transmission. Your confusion and humiliation are not accidental; they're a feature, not a bug, of the PR strategy. For it is only by
reconciling contradictions that power can be retained indefinitely, as
Orwell taught us.

During the covid pandemic, several terms of disparagement were repeatedly deployed against anyone who questioned the favored policies. These
phrases functioned not to illuminate but to halt the possibility of critical
thought or rational debate. They formed part of the elaborate system to
forbid certain questions. These terms included, among others, *covid denier*,
anti-vax, and *conspiracy theorist*. I anticipate that some critics will mischar-
acterize this book using these and similar terms—ready-made cognitive

shortcuts that save critics the trouble of reading the book or critically engaging my evidence or arguments.

A brief comment on each of these may be helpful to illustrate how these terms function analogously to Orwell's Newspeak. The first term, "covid denier" (or "pandemic denier"), requires little critical analysis. Those who sling this charge at any skeptic of our pandemic response recklessly equate covid with the Holocaust, a move which suggests the degree to which antisemitism continues to infect discourse on both the Right and the Left. We need not detain ourselves with additional commentary on this thought-stopping, mind-numbing phrase. I have yet to meet a person who denied the existence of covid or ignored the fact that the virus has tragically killed too many people.

The epithet "anti-vax," deployed to characterize anyone who raises questions about the mass vaccination campaign or the safety and efficacy of covid vaccines, functions similarly as a conversation stopper rather than an accurately descriptive label. Those who were injured by covid vaccines and tried to speak publicly about their serious vaccine-adverse effects, for example, were routinely pummeled with the anti-vax label, begging the obvious question: Why would people who were anti-vaccine take a vaccine that injured them in the first place?

When people ask me whether I am anti-vax because I legally challenged vaccine mandates, I can only respond that the question makes little sense: it's like asking whether I am "pro-medication" or "anti-medication." For any sensible physician, the answer can only be contingent and nuanced: Which medication, for which patient or patient population, under what circumstances, and for what indications? There is clearly no such thing as a medication—or a vaccine—that's always good for everyone in every circumstance all the time. That's not how human biology and medicine work.

The term "conspiracy theorist" requires a bit more commentary. Giorgio Agamben noted that the indiscriminate deployment of this term during the pandemic demonstrated a surprising historical ignorance.[13] Anyone familiar with history knows that the stories historians tell frequently retrace and reconstruct the actions of individuals, groups, and factions working together in common purpose to achieve their goals using all available means. That is, history is replete with stories of how people deliberately *conspire* and thereby change the course of historical events. He mentions three examples from among thousands in the historical record.

In 415 BC, Alcibiades deployed his influence and money to convince the Athenians to embark on an expedition to Sicily. This venture turned out disastrously and marked the end of Athenian supremacy. In retaliation, his enemies hired false witnesses and conspired against Alcibiades to condemn him to death.

In 1799 Napoleon Bonaparte violated his oath of fidelity to the French Republic's constitution, overthrowing the directory in a coup, assuming full dictatorial powers, and putting an end to the French Revolution. In the days leading up to this, Napoleon had met with coconspirators to fine-tune their strategy against the anticipated opposition of the Republic's Council of Five Hundred. The entire operation was strategically planned and carefully coordinated down to the last detail.

Closer to our own day, in October 1922, twenty-five thousand Italian Fascists marched on Rome and took power. Leading up to this event, Mussolini prepared the march with three close collaborators and initiated contacts with the prime minister and powerful figures from the Italian business world. Some historians maintain that Mussolini even secretly met with the king to explore possible allegiances. The Fascists had carefully rehearsed their occupation of Rome by conducting a military occupation of Ancona two months prior.

Countless other examples of conspiracies that changed history—from the murder of Julius Caesar to the Bolshevik Revolution—will readily occur to any student of history. In all these instances, individuals gathered in groups or parties to strategize goals and tactics, anticipate obstacles, and then act resolutely to achieve their aims using all the means—licit or illicit—at their disposal. Of course, this does not mean that we must always resort to conspiracies to explain historical events. But as Agamben writes, "Anyone who labelled a historian who tried to reconstruct in detail the plots that triggered such events as a 'conspiracy theorist' would most definitely be demonstrating their own ignorance, if not idiocy."[14]

Event 201 and the other pandemic war-game scenarios described in the opening chapter are merely contemporary examples of powerful people and their affiliated organizations coordinating their efforts, jointly pursuing their objectives, and collectively trying to realize their goals by all available means. Likewise with the individuals and organizations we will encounter later in this chapter, whose aims and actions before and during the pandemic are well attested and clearly documented, if we just take them at their own word. By 2022, in the wake of new revelations about the lab-leak hypothesis, NIH funding of gain-of-function research at the Wuhan Institute of Virology, vaccine safety issues willfully suppressed, and coordinated media and government smear and censorship campaigns against dissident scientific voices, it seemed the only difference between a conspiracy theory and credible news was about six months.

Anyone who worried about "the Great Reset" in 2019 was accused of peddling a conspiracy theory—that is, until World Economic Forum (WEF) founder and executive chairman Klaus Schwab, with coauthor Thierry Malleret, published a book in 2020 laying out the WEF agenda with the helpful title *COVID-19: The Great Reset*.[15] If this is a conspiracy, the conspirators' game plan is not exactly top secret, even if it's presented in Schwab's turgid style of leaden prose. The book is an appallingly written tome filled with foggy notions alternating with grandiose assertions. The Great Reset agenda described therein is nothing if not ambitious.

In their own words, in the wake of covid, "a new world will emerge, the contours of which are for us to both imagine and to draw." Things will never return to normal, for "nothing will ever return to the 'broken' sense of normalcy that prevailed prior to the crisis because the coronavirus pandemic marks a fundamental inflection point in our global trajectory." Schwab opines that the radical changes will be of such enormous consequence that we may speak of a "before coronavirus" (BC) and "after coronavirus" (AC)—such are the biblical proportions of our present turning point. The coming changes, Schwab explains, "will shape a 'new normal' radically different from the one we will be progressively leaving behind. Many of our beliefs and assumptions about what the world could or should look like will be shattered in the process."[16]

Recall in this context our discussion of the myth of a radical revolutionary break with all previous history that characterized the twentieth-century totalitarian ideologies. We hear strong echoes of this in Schwab's rhetoric. Schwab's proposal imagines "macro resets" in the economic, societal, geopolitical, environmental, and technological domains, as well as "micro resets" in industry and business and "individual resets" that include "redefining our humanness." Getting down to specifics, the immediate political changes Schwab foresees include familiar bromides such as open borders but travel restrictions for otherwise legal border crossings, higher taxes and the expansion of government, working-class dependence upon a welfare state, and supply chain disruptions. It also includes proposals for carbon allowances, along with the digital surveillance infrastructure necessary to monitor people's movements and purchases, as sketched in this chapter's opening hypothetical scenario.

Schwab considers proposing periodic lockdowns to reduce carbon emissions, but eventually concludes that the results from lockdowns alone would still be insufficient to address the scope of the climate change problem. More than this, he argues that we need "a radical and major systemic change in how we produce the energy needed to function and structural changes in our consumption behavior."[17] He opines that in the future governments will most likely "decide that it's in the best interest of society to rewrite some of the rules of the game and permanently increase their role."[18] The entire social contract, he argues, will need to be redefined in the wake of the covid pandemic. As I said, the program is nothing if not ambitious.

Schwab—along with his coconspirators and associates at the WEF—is not so much an evil genius manipulating the levers of power from a smoke-filled resort room in Davos. He is more like a cartoonish mascot, a garish distillation and personification of a widely shared ideology and an ambitious agenda embraced by many corporate, tech, finance, and political power brokers with globalist pretentions. That the institutions and interests of these elites often interlock, that they meet regularly in Davos, a resort town in the Swiss Alps, to plan and coordinate their efforts, should come as no surprise. WEF globalists are far from alone: many who don't get invited to the Davos parties have their own roles to play and dutifully take their cues from their cultural overlords. For their part, universities and their administrators, along with scores of media talking heads, readily and willingly serve among the ranks of those Lenin (rather indelicately) called "useful idiots" for advancing this agenda.

The WEF is representative, and we can take that word literally. It is a nominally nonprofit trade organization representing, according to its website, its one thousand member companies. These companies are global enterprises, typically with more than five trillion U.S. dollars in turnover—the biggest of the corporate big dogs. Their CEOs—an elite set of oligarchs Samuel Huntington referred to as "Davos Man"—constitute the 1 percent of the 1 percent of the 1 percent. The WEF functions to advance its members' interests, not to make the world better, whatever the rhetoric generated by its PR armies and obsequious journalists eager for access to power.

Our ruling class saw in covid an opportunity to revolutionize society. Recall how the phrase "the new normal" emerged almost immediately in the initial weeks of the pandemic. In the first month Anthony Fauci suggested that perhaps we would never again go back to shaking hands. Really? Never? The WHO's director general Tedros explained this clearly, echoing Schwab: "I want to be straight with you: There will be no return to the old normal for the foreseeable future."

Eighty years ago, C. S. Lewis foresaw the coming oligarchic technocracy in a book appropriately titled *The Abolition of Man*. I consider this short, deceptively simple book to be among the most important and prescient works of the twentieth century. In the closing chapter, Lewis makes the following prediction and poses the following question:

> The final stage is come when Man by eugenics, by pre-natal conditioning, and by an education and propaganda based on a perfect applied psychology, has obtained full control over himself. Human nature will be the last part of Nature to surrender to Man. The battle will then be won. We shall . . . be henceforth free to make our species whatever we wish it to be. The battle will indeed be won. But who, precisely, will have won it?[19]

Who, indeed?

The New Lords of the World

Given the staggering failures of our pandemic policies, many of which were abandoned in early 2022 following the omicron variant wake-up call, we might wonder: Why has there still been virtually no reckoning with those failures? Where is the serious, and very necessary, postmortem on the pandemic? Perhaps a rigorous retrospective critique of our pandemic policies has not happened because many of the key policies were not really about the virus in the first place. They were adopted with other aims in mind, and they successfully served these other interests, mostly financial and political. The biomedical security state serves interests other than public health.

Our covid response amounted to a class war. Rolling lockdowns plunged people into poverty worldwide while the shrunken middle class was hit by skyrocketing inflation. According to data from the Federal Reserve, following the pandemic the top 1 percent of U.S. earners have more wealth than the entire middle class. The richest 10 percent now own 90 percent of stocks.[20] By October 2021 the combined wealth of billionaires had risen by $2.1 trillion during the pandemic, a 70 percent increase that brought their collective worth to $5 trillion—roughly the GDP of Japan, the world's third-largest economy. Meanwhile, their philanthropic contributions fell to their lowest in more than a decade, at a time when an estimated 500 million people fell into poverty.[21]

The federal CARES Act bailed out many large monopolistic firms with little regulation or oversight of how the money was spent. Airline executives, for example, used this taxpayer money to give themselves bonuses while laying off tens of thousands of employees.[22] In 2020, as the Fed provided enormous purchases of corporate debt and securities, "millions of people filed for unemployment, [and] nearly 1 in 4 households experienced food insecurity," journalist Alex Gutentag explained. "The result was an estimated loss of $1.3 trillion in household wealth for American workers. Meanwhile, U.S. billionaires gained $1 trillion."[23] By June 2020 more than 400,000 small businesses had closed, with additional closures continuing through the second half of that year. By the end of May 2021, there were 40 percent fewer small businesses nationwide than at the beginning of 2020.[24]

The lockdown-induced carnage was even worse internationally, particularly in developing nations. An estimated 140 million people, at minimum, were added to the number of people on the edge of starvation, and this is likely to worsen. An additional 70,000 children died of malaria in 2020 compared to the previous year—mostly because they could not access clinics when they had a fever or could not get the necessary medications due to lockdown-induced supply chain problems. Tuberculosis and HIV rates also rose dramatically. School closures crippled the ability of countries to rise out of poverty: UNICEF estimated an additional 10 million girls will be forced into child marriage due to school closures and poverty. Also, according to their calculations, in six South Asian countries in 2020 an estimated 228,000 infants and children died and an additional 400,000 teenage pregnancies occurred due to lockdown-related disruptions.

Social distancing encouraged citizens to view friends and neighbors as potential threats, and thus as the villains of the pandemic. We were directed instead to see experts, technocrats, and corporations as the heroes of the pandemic.[25] These "heroes," not coincidentally, made record profits. This two-tiered society was further cemented in 2021 with the introduction of vaccine mandates and passports, which created a permanent underclass banished from professional life and excluded from economic activity. The passport system disproportionately impacted and excluded poor and working-class people, especially people of color. As Gutentag summarized: "This is not an unforced error or a good policy idea implemented poorly. It is an economic agenda disguised as a health protocol."[26]

It is not difficult to identify the global financial interests that drove our failed pandemic response. Many of the key players gather with select celebrities, heads of state, and journalists every year in Davos. We may be tempted to see the WEF and its leaders as a coterie of supervillains pulling the levers of power. After all, we like it when the bad guys are identifiable. But as I already suggested, it is more accurate to see Schwab and company simply as *visible distillations* of ideologies embraced by many of our global financial elites.

A tree is known by its fruits. During the lockdowns we saw the largest upward transfer of wealth in human history. WEF members were massively enriched by our pandemic policies, while millions of less fortunate souls were plunged into poverty and misery. Nothing trickled down from the top to relieve the destitution of the masses. The cash that flowed to Davos Man stayed in Davos Man's pocket. The meager resources at the bottom, and the hard-won resources in the middle, were vacuumed upwards, all the way up to the peak of the socioeconomic pyramid. This trend started before the pandemic and achieved record velocity during covid. Davos Man helped craft the pandemic rules in his own interests, orchestrating a staggering, world-historical scheme of larceny.

Peter Goodman, the global economics correspondent for the *New York Times* and a man of the Left, documented the gruesome details of this organized theft in part II of his book *Davos Man: How Billionaires*

Devoured the World, under the heading, "Profiteering Off a Pandemic."[27] In the wake of the pandemic, the richest ten people in the world now have combined wealth greater than the poorest eighty-five countries combined. Pause for a moment and try to wrap your mind around that. This outcome was neither accidental nor caused by a virus. It was driven by specific policies that our elites orchestrated and that we accepted. Let us not be deceived: the devil dances in Davos.

The WEF cast of characters represent and publicly articulate the aspirations of Big Tech corporate behemoths, enormous worldwide finance firms like BlackRock and Blackstone, globalist NGOs and foundations, and other powerful moneyed interests. Many of these firms have more capital than they know what to do with; what they want now is power. Their endgame is corporatism: the merging of corporate interests and government, or more accurately, the control of governing institutions by corporate interests. Naturally, the heads of state gathered at Davos aim to be the ones using the corporations to advance their political agendas.

Both sides deploy the euphemistic language of "public-private partnerships" and "stakeholder capitalism" to sell their microwaved model of corporatism. But as Andrew Stuttaford remarked, corporatism is often "framed to look like cooperation, but is all too frequently under-pinned by coercion,"[28] because it necessarily entails that government will intervene more in the affairs of business and business will intervene more in the affairs of government. Concepts like public-private partnerships can sound benign until you scratch beneath the surface.

For example, in 2019 the UK government announced its partnership with the WEF to develop industrial, business, and economic regulations for the future. The British government indicated its commitment to supporting a regulatory environment created and managed by global corporations, which in turn would be regulated by the same regulations they had designed.[29] This model of an industry capturing the very government agencies that are supposed to regulate that industry is clearly not confined to pharma's capture of the CDC and FDA, which we explored previously.

Before we unthinkingly embrace the WEF's and the WHO's proposals for public-private partnerships, it's worth recalling that Mussolini's definition of Fascism coincided perfectly with the definition of corporatism—the merger of state and corporate power.

Note carefully the language introducing global public-private partnerships in the 2005 WHO document *Connecting for Health*, which expounds upon the UN's Millennium Development Goals for Health:

> These changes occurred in a world of revised expectations about the role of government: that the public sector has neither the financial nor the institutional resources to meet their challenges, and that a mix of public and private resources is required. . . . Building a global culture of security and cooperation is vital. . . . The beginnings of a global health infrastructure are already in place. . . . Information and communication technologies have opened opportunities for change in health, with or without policy-makers leading the way. . . . Governments can create an enabling environment, and invest in equity, access and innovation.[30]

You read that correctly: the WHO expects that governments will have a *revised* role, given that they have neither the financial nor institutional resources to meet public health challenges. Private resources will be required to build a "global culture of security" and the needed "global health infrastructure." This will happen "*with or without* policy-makers'"—that is, duly elected officials—stamp of approval. Information and communication technologies have created opportunities for changes in health management, which unelected private commercial interests will exploit. The document explains that, in their diminished roles, governments can still create an "enabling environment" through taxation and increased government debt while allowing corporate leaders to manage the details of policy and implementation for the new global health empire.

This would sound like aspirational bloviation—the same impenetrable bureaucratese dialect used by UN agencies for decades in countless reports—if not for the fact that this model was actually implemented globally during covid. Nothing else could have so rapidly advanced this agenda like a pandemic. Perhaps this explains why the WEF helped fund many of the pandemic war-gaming exercises described in the first chapter. Echoing Rahm Emanuel's advice to "never let a crisis go to waste," Schwab and his coauthor Thierry Malleret saw covid as an "opportunity [that] can be seized." If the past five centuries in Europe and America have taught us anything, they assert, it is this: "Acute crises contribute to boosting the power of the state. It's always been the case and there is no reason why it should be different with the COVID-19 pandemic."[31]

Lockdowns accomplished exactly what the WEF and its global affiliates wanted, eliminating competition for monopolistic global firms by closing small businesses and vacuuming wealth upwards. Schwab argues that rather than just fixing market failures when they arise, governments should "move towards actively shaping and creating markets that deliver sustainable and inclusive growth."[32] We already witnessed this kind of corporatism, in which governments rewrote the rules of the game and created markets for business, with covid vaccines: in exchange for granting pharma protection from all liability and guaranteeing an enormous market for its product via mandates, the state acquired a vehicle to expand its coercive powers over the bodies of citizens.

In this arrangement corporate stakeholders become what Michael Rectenwald calls "governmentalities," which are "otherwise 'private' organizations wielded as state apparatuses, with no obligation to answer to pesky constituents." Furthermore, as Rectenwald notes, "since these corporations are multinational, the state essentially becomes global, whether or not a 'one-world government' is ever formalized."[33] With this form of corporatism, the state's reach is extended through the deployment of corporate assets—a win-win for the favored corporation and its government cronies, a lose-lose for everyone else.

Agamben dubbed these current microwaved forms of corporatism "capitalism in its communist variation." He explains that this model "unites an extremely rapid development of production with a totalitarian political regime."[34] China has taken the lead role in advancing this model, especially during the pandemic, where rapid development and production were managed by a totalitarian state. Many observers in the West mistakenly assumed that the "state capitalism" established in supposedly communist countries like China represented a form of capitalism specifically adapted for economically backward countries. They incorrectly predicted that once this form of capitalism had served its temporary function, it was destined to become obsolete, giving way to free and open democracies. On the contrary, China demonstrated that capitalism and freedom are not necessarily coterminous. Instead, with some technological upgrades, communist capitalism emerged during the pandemic as "the ruling principle of the current phase of globalized capitalism."

We can foresee a conflict between an ascendant capitalism in its communist variation (a form of fascism, according to the strict definition of that word) and the old capitalism characteristic of bourgeois Western democracies. The outcome of this conflict remains uncertain. For my part I worry that this tension may inescapably escalate to armed conflict between China and the West, though I pray it does not come to that. It is also possible that communist capitalism will prevail without the force of arms. "What is certain, however," Agamben writes, "is that the new regime will combine the most inhumane aspects of capitalism with the most atrocious aspects of state communism, combining the extreme alienation of relations between people with an unprecedented social control."[35] Communist capitalism is the economic form of the rising biomedical security state.

Ongoing states of emergency will accelerate this process. Schwab and Malleret cite Joseph Stigliz to explain that funding to the public sector must increase because we can anticipate moving from one crisis to the next: "Even as we emerge from this crisis, we should be aware that some other crisis surely lurks around the corner. We can't predict what the next one will look like—other than it will look different from the last."[36] There you have it, straight from the source. It's not a prophecy; it's a plan.

The WEF made waves last year by posting on its website the slogan, "You will own nothing. And you will be happy." Although the page was later deleted, the indelible impression remained: it provided a clear and simple description of the future envisioned by Davos Man. As the WEF savants predict, at the last stage of this development, we will find ourselves in a rent-only/subscription-only economy, where nothing really belongs to us. Picture the Uberization of everything.

To get a sense of this future, imagine the world as an Amazon warehouse writ large: a mandarin caste of digital virtuosos will call the shots from behind screens, directing the masses below with the aid of ever more refined algorithmic specificity. The prophetic Aldous Huxley foresaw this "brave new world" in his 1932 novel. These changes will challenge not only our political, economic, and medical institutions and structures; they will challenge our notions of what it means to be human. This is precisely what their advocates celebrate, as we will see later in this chapter.

Capitalism in its communist variation, facilitated by the corporatist arrangements of public-private partnerships, is well suited for carrying out the desired convergence of existing and emerging fields. This biological-digital convergence envisioned by the WEF and its members will blend big data, artificial intelligence, machine learning, genetics, nanotechnology, and robotics. Schwab refers to this as the Fourth Industrial Revolution, which will follow and build upon the first three—mechanical, electrical, and digital. The transhumanists, whom we will meet shortly, have been dreaming of just such a merging of the physical, digital, and biological worlds for at least a few decades. Now, however, their visions are poised to become our reality.

• • •

The WHO is likewise pursuing new models to augment its own power and facilitate centralized control by unelected bureaucrats. The

WHO recently announced plans for an international pandemic treaty tied to a digital passport and digital ID system. Meeting in December 2021, in a special session for only the second time since the WHO's founding in 1948, the Health Assembly of the WHO adopted a single resolution titled "The World Together," approving plans for the treaty.[37] The WHO hopes to finalize the treaty by 2024. It aims to shift governing authority, now reserved to sovereign states, to the WHO during a pandemic.

This will be accomplished by legally binding member states to the WHO's revised International Health Regulations.[38] In January 2022 the Biden administration submitted proposed amendments to the 2005 International Health Regulations (IHR), which bind all 193 UN member states. The WHO director general accepted and forwarded the United States' proposed amendments to other member states. Unlike amendments to our Constitution, these will not require a two-thirds vote of our Senate, but a simple majority of the UN member states. Most of the public is wholly unaware of these proposed changes to international law, which will impact the national sovereignty of all member states, including the United States.

The proposed amendments include the following changes. First, the WHO will no longer need to consult with the state or attempt to obtain verification from the state where an event of concern (for example, a new outbreak) is allegedly occurring before acting on such reports (Article 9.1). In addition to the authority to determine a public health emergency of *international* concern under Article 12, the WHO will be granted additional powers to determine a public health emergency of *regional* concern, as well as a new category referred to as an intermediate health alert.

The relevant state no longer needs to agree with the WHO director general's determination that an event constitutes a public health emergency of international concern. A new Emergency Committee will be constituted at the WHO, which the director general will consult in lieu of the state within whose territory the public health emergency has occurred, to declare the emergency over. The amendments will also give regional directors within the WHO, rather than elected representatives of the relevant state, the legal authority to declare a public health emergency of regional concern.[39]

When an event does not meet criteria for a public health emergency of international or regional concern but the WHO director general believes it requires heightened awareness and a potential international public health response, he may determine at any time to issue an "intermediate public health alert" to states and to consult the WHO's Emergency Committee. The criterion for this intermediate category is simple fiat: an event meets the criterion when "the Director-General has determined it requires heightened international awareness and a potential international public health response."[40] This tautological definition means that it is one when the director general says it is one.

Through these amendments, the WHO, with the support of the United States, appears to be responding to roadblocks that China erected in the early days of covid. That is a legitimate concern, since the Chinese Communist Party's attempt to cover up the initial outbreak delayed the response and arguably allowed the virus to spread when it might have been regionally contained. But the net effect of the proposed amendments is a shift of power away from sovereign states, ours included, to unelected bureaucrats at the WHO. This is not a wise solution to a problem created by an authoritarian regime. The thrust of every one of the proposed changes is toward increasingly centralized powers delegated to the WHO and away from sovereign member states.

Leslyn Lewis, a member of the Canadian Parliament and lawyer with international experience, has warned that the treaty would allow the WHO to determine unilaterally what constitutes a pandemic and declare when a pandemic is occurring. Rather than permitting regional responses to local realities on the ground, "we would end up with a one-size-fits-all approach for the entire world," she cautioned. Furthermore, under the proposed WHO plan, pandemics need not be limited to infectious diseases and could include, for example, a declared obesity crisis.[41]

In what is probably more consequential than even these IHR changes, the WHO will also create a permanent new bureaucracy responsible for the ongoing monitoring of pandemics. This entity will need to routinely find and declare outbreaks and pandemics to justify its continued existence—even though historically we typically have only three or four pandemics in a century, and only one of these is typically serious and sustained. Prior to the Spanish flu in 1918, most pandemics like the Black Plague were cause by bacterial illnesses, which are no longer a threat with the advent of antibiotics. Viral pandemics are relatively rare occurrences and are typically not very serious.

As part of this plan—and this represents one of the corporatist "public-private partnership" elements—the WHO already contracted with Germany-based Deutsche Telekom subsidiary T-Systems to develop a global vaccine passport system, with plans to link every person on the planet to a digital ID. As Garrett Mehl, head of the WHO's Department of Digital Health and Innovation, explained, "The WHO's gateway service also serves as a bridge between regional systems. It can also be used as part of future vaccination campaigns and home-based records."[42] The WHO's digital system of biomedical surveillance and control will be mandatory, transnational, and operated by unelected bureaucrats operating in a captured NGO that has already badly bungled the covid pandemic response.

I do not want to give the impression that the WHO is an agency bent on world domination; it is far too incompetent for such a grandiose task. On the contrary the WHO is an enormous global bureaucracy that mostly responds to the will of its funders. As we have seen, most of its funding now comes from private sources, not member nations. Unlike contributions from governments, private contributions come with highly specified projects the money is earmarked to fund, right down to specifying exactly who will be involved in the funded projects. The nonprofit and for-profit private nongovernmental entities funneling money to the WHO will be the ones pulling the strings, with the WHO acting as a useful public international instrument to advance their private agendas.

Biodigital Surveillance

Flying from LAX to Boston recently, as I walked toward security, I was intercepted by a saleswoman asking if I wanted to skip the security line. Intrigued, I invited her to tell me more. She shuttled me over to the CLEAR electronic kiosk and explained how the product worked. For only $180 a year I could skip long lines at airports, sporting events, and other large gatherings. As CLEAR advertises, "Instead of using traditional ID documents, CLEAR uses your eyes and face to confirm it's really you." In fact, the system uses not just an iris scan and facial recognition, but other biometrics such as fingerprints, tied to demographic data you voluntarily hand over, and a link to your credit score (read the fine print on the consent checkbox). CLEAR also has a Health Pass that stores proof of vaccination, negative covid tests, and health surveys. The company currently partners with Delta and United Airlines, a network of merchants called Partnership for New York City, and many sports venues.[43]

Plans for digital IDs have been in the works for several years, but they required a pandemic to gain traction. ID2020 is a nonprofit alliance founded in 2016 with seed money from Microsoft, Accenture, PricewaterhouseCoopers, the Rockefeller Foundation, Cisco, and Gavi (a vaccine alliance founded by the Gates Foundation). The stated mission of ID2020 is to provide digital identities for all people worldwide by 2030: these will be tied to fingerprints and other biometric data like iris scans, demographic information, medical records, and data on education, travel, financial transactions, and bank accounts.

Almost two years before covid, ID2020 published an article in March 2018 titled "Immunization: An Entry Point for Digital Identity," which argued that "immunization poses a huge opportunity to scale digital identity." The article noted cumbersome inefficiencies with paper immunization records and delineated how health challenges in developing nations could be leveraged as the pretext for implementing digital IDs.[44]

The year before, in 2017, Seth Berkley, CEO of Gavi, published a piece in *Nature* with the title "Immunization Needs a Technology

Boost," which made the same argument: to achieve 100 percent vaccination rates in underdeveloped nations we need digital IDs for tracking them.[45] At the 2018 WEF meeting in Davos, Gavi announced digital identity as the focus of its new INFUSE program (Innovation for Uptake, Scale and Equity in Immunization—got to love these euphemistic acronyms). The ID2020 article attempts to frame the benefits of this system as follows:

> Because immunization is conducted in infancy, providing children with a digital child health card would give them a unique, portable digital identity early in life. And as children grow, their digital child health card can be used to access secondary services, such as primary school, or ease the process of obtaining alternative credentials. Effectively the child health card becomes the first step in establishing a legal, broadly recognized identity.[46]

This may at first glance sound sensible. However, consider the corollary of this system: if an impoverished family does not accept the health NGO's preferred interventions for their children, these children may not be provided any other opportunity to establish a "legal, broadly recognized identity" necessary to access things like primary school. In other words, you are literally nobody until you are vaccinated.

Just before the pandemic broke, in September 2019, ID2020 partnered with Gavi and begin putting this plan into action, launching a biometrics-based digital identity program for newborn infants in Bangladesh using vaccination as leverage. The government of Bangladesh willingly embraced this program.[47] When the pandemic began, ID2020 pivoted immediately to fold digital identification into covid testing and other pandemic measures.

Using biometrics for everyday transactions routinizes these technologies. We are conditioning children to accept biometric verification as a matter of course. For example, face IDs are now used in multiple school districts to expedite the movement of students through school lunch lines. Until recently, biometrics such as fingerprints were used only for high-security purposes—when charging someone with a crime, for example, or when notarizing an important document. Today, routine biometric verification for things from mobile phones to lunch lines gets young people used to the idea that *their bodies are tools used in transactions.* We are instrumentalizing the body in unconscious and subtle, but nonetheless powerful, ways.

India's biometric ID system, Aadhaar, is the largest on the planet, with 1.3 billion digital IDs issued covering 92 percent of the population. It requires India's citizens to submit their photograph, iris scan, and fingerprints to qualify for social services, benefits, compensation, scholarships, legal entitlements, and nutrition programs. According to an article in the *Financial Times*, "Indian media has reported several cases of cardless individuals starving to death because they could not access benefits to which they were entitled." Some critics argue the Indian Aadhaar system "has largely failed to fulfil its original promise of improving welfare and now acts as a tool for social exclusion and corporate influence."[48]

During the pandemic, the city of Varanasi in northern India installed CCTV cameras citywide that utilize automated facial recognition, as part of its "smart city" enterprise. Authorities claim the system will only be used to track suspected criminals or find missing children. Oh, yes . . . and for contact tracing. The temptation to additional mission creep will likely prove impossible to resist.

In the United Kingdom, the South Wales police department has pioneered the use of facial recognition technology, deploying it at public events on about fifty occasions from 2017 to 2019. The Philippines announced a similar program in 2020, with facial recognition cameras capable of night vision. Manila city mayor Isko Moreno bragged that faces and plate numbers will be seen "even in the darkest portion of the city."[49] The panopticon never blinks. Or sleeps.

The world already contains over one billion surveillance cameras. While half are in China, the United States now has almost as many cameras per capita (1 camera per 4.6 people) as China (1 per 4.1). After the Chinese cities of Taiyuan and Wuxi, the city with the most surveillance cameras per capita is London. Both the United Kingdom and the United States are now heavily investing in facial recognition technologies, and cities such as Detroit, Orlando, and Washington, D.C., are testing the use of facial recognition video feeds in policing and security.[50]

Those with economic interests in creating markets for their products (whether vaccines, digital surveillance hardware and software, or harvested data) will continue to deploy the carrots and sticks of access to medical care and other services to strong-arm acceptance of digital IDs in underdeveloped nations. In developed nations they will initially use a velvet glove approach of nudges, selling digital IDs as conveniences and time-saving measures that will be hard for many to turn down, such as skipping long TSA security lines at airports. The privacy risks, including the possibility for constant surveillance and data harvesting, will fade into the background when you're about to miss your flight if you can't skip to the front of the line.

But as Nick Corbishley points out, decisions made in the moment may carry long-term negative consequences: "If biometric data is hacked, there is no way of undoing the damage. You cannot change or cancel your iris, fingerprint, or DNA like you can change a password or cancel your credit card."[51] Unless we collectively decline to participate in this new social experiment, digital IDs—tied to private demographic, financial, location, movement, and biometric data—will become mechanisms for bulk data harvesting and tracking of populations around the globe. Digital IDs are inextricably bound up with the biomedical security state.

● ● ●

Related developments involve increased digital control of currency and exchange. During the first year of the covid pandemic China released the e-Yuan, a digital currency controlled by China's central banks under the thumb of Beijing. For those unfamiliar with the cryptocurrency world, it's important to distinguish decentralized currencies like Bitcoin from central bank digital currencies (CBDCs) like China's e-Yuan. This distinction is crucial because the latter, CBDCs, are not really currencies at all, as I will explain in a moment.

The International Monetary Fund (IMF) is now promoting CBDCs, especially for lower-income countries and emerging markets. The IMF admits that there are downsides: privacy may be compromised, and digital payment companies are increasingly capturing and monetizing consumer data. Digital currencies are also at risk from cyberattacks, outages, technical glitches, fraud risks, and faulty algorithms. More concerningly, the IMF also notes that the legal status of digital currencies is unclear: Are they money, bank deposits, securities, commodities, or something else entirely?[52]

If the government through the central bank gives you a tax credit in the form of CBDC, the government or central bank can put restrictions on how and when you spend it. For example, the government could specify that you need to spend your tax credit in the next eighteen months on clean energy, or could prohibit you from spending it on a particular list of disfavored industries or products, or whatever. If you don't spend it within the allotted time frame, the government or central bank could simply make the "money" disappear.

Thus, what you have in your digital wallet is not really money, not in fact a wholly fungible asset that belongs to you until you spend it, as currency has traditionally functioned. What you have is a kind of temporary voucher. Once these currencies are tied to measures of social credit—such as vaccine status, ratings and markers of compliance, or proof of socially sanctioned behaviors—private economic transactions will be subjected to unprecedented external monitoring and control. No exchange of money, however small, will really be private and free of external influence.

With central bank digital currencies, buying and selling would become "closer to a form of bondage than to monetary exchange," in Alex Gutentag's words. "Instead of sums of money, a [CBDC] bank account would come to represent tokens that could be turned on and off based on good or bad behavior." This is among the reasons that several of our pandemic measures were so politically consequential. "The vaccine passport and the crackdown against Covid dissent served as a test run for this model," as Gutentag explains. "But the inability of unvaccinated people to access a gym or a bar will pale in comparison to the types of punishments that can be meted out through such a system, not just for members of a political opposition, but for their families or anyone who dares to help them."[53]

Recall the Canadian government's freezing the bank accounts of the truckers and their benefactors. Imagine that kind of power expanded by orders of magnitude. With CBDCs the government can track every one of your transactions down to the last penny. These "currencies" therefore become a massive data-gathering mechanism when tied to your digital ID via the app used for market transactions. Extensive research by Shoshana Zuboff on our current system of surveillance capitalism has clearly shown that your data is now a product to be sold.[54] Or more accurately, you are the product. Or even more accurately, you are the raw material from which the product is made.

This system dehumanizes people not only by diminishing their financial freedom, but also by reifying and commoditizing them. Once fully realized, this surveillance system will offer unprecedented mechanisms of control, allowing the regime to be maintained against any form of resistance. This technocratic dream would entrench the most "conservative" system the world has ever known—in the sense that it could maintain itself against any form of opposition through monopolistic technological and economic power. The suppression of dissent will happen in large part through the system's financial controls. Try to resist or step outside the system's strictures and the doors to markets will simply close. This means that once this system is in place, it could prove almost impossible to overthrow.

This system will be implemented and maintained by an oligarchic class, a "new alliance guided by a technocratic elite that occupies the main political, cultural, economic, and educational institutions," as political theorist Patrick Deneen describes. He explains that this new class "arises in the name of the proletariat, but quickly assumes power through its abilities to wield the tools of the technocracy. Increasingly, this class finds itself at odds with the proletariat that it was purportedly empowered to liberate."[55] Instead of leading to greater economic equality, the system will only further entrench the power of the technocratic bourgeoisie and their elite overlords, exacerbating class disparities and further disempowering the working class and the poor.

Deneen predicts that "traditional forms of life, which offer some resistance to concentrations of power, would be relentlessly targeted by the supposed agents of liberation." This scientistic-technocratic system provides an illusion of individual liberation via rapid change, but will in fact be built on a deeper foundation of rigid control. It would, in his words, "cement an order governed by titanic economic, social, and political organizations that would provide the patina of liberation while controlling resources, finance, political power, and (today) data."[56] In the wake of these transformations, the old definitions of right and left will be rendered obsolete: we will end up with an unbreakable alliance between the cultural left and the technocratic right—communist capitalism, to borrow Agamben's term.

The window for opposing this system's entrenchment is short and rapidly closing.

• • •

The Chinese digital Yuan has already taken their social-credit system international: it reaches across borders to any investors who utilize it. The circulation of the Chinese cryptocurrency is controlled by the state, and only authorized brokers and banks can initially sell it. Early indications suggest that investors are buying, as Yahoo Finance recently reported: "After the e-Yuan announcement, Chinese technology stocks have been steadily reaching new record heights with Foreigners recently spending over $26.99 Billion on technology stocks listed in Shenzhen stock exchange. All of this provides great returns for both e-Yuan and Chinese technology stock investors."[57]

At the recent Beijing Olympic Games, the Chinese Communist Party forced participants to download and enroll in its e-Yuan app and use it for all purchases while in Beijing. The CCP can obviously force this on the Chinese population, but this move at the Olympics proved it could also force it on foreign nationals from dozens of other countries. The party's goals in this global rollout included not only reducing its dependence on the foreign dollar, but also exporting the Chinese tech stack into everyone in the developed world.

The e-Yuan software is not just a payment app, but an app that tracks all your identifying data (name, social security number, eventually biometric and health data), your location at any moment, all your financial transactions and accounts, and so on. It allows a direct line from the Chinese government to the individual—whether native or foreign—outside the purview of law enforcement, banking regulator oversight, or national privacy safeguards. Suppose, for example, there's a U.S. government employee short on cash from serious gambling debts: the app can extract that information for use by the CCP—useful leverage for Chinese foreign intelligence. The centrally controlled digital currency provides an access point to corrupt anyone who is corruptible and to blackmail anyone who falls. It will function as a tool for digital export of the Chinese Communist Party's authoritarianism, coercion, and bribery that's long been par for the course for this regime.

China is not alone in its interest in central bank digital currencies. Seventy percent of other nations are contemplating launching their own CBDCs. The feds are now considering a digital dollar, which would bring this system to the United States.[58] India announced recently it plans to create a digital rupee. Jamaica, Zambia, and Kenya will likely follow suit. The UK government recently signed a contract with Deloitte to develop a new digital ID system, and Canada plans to roll out digital IDs at the urging of the Canadian Bankers Association.[59] There is a concurrent push to eliminate all cash transactions—cash being one of the last vestiges of freedom, privacy, and anonymity—supported by companies rolling out digital IDs. Clearly, digital IDs and CBDCs are designed to operate hand in glove. Both are central tools of the biomedical security state.

In summary, both information exchange and monetary exchange will be monitored and controlled with digital ID–enabled social-credit systems, which reward conformity with inclusion in society and the market and punish nonconformity with exclusion. In China one of the sticks used to punish those with dings on their social-credit score is the inability to board a train or plane. It's worth noticing that Canadian and European vaccine passport systems used the very same punishment for the unvaccinated.

As this system develops, an increasingly wide range of human activities, from reproduction to religion, could come under surveillance and technological control. Vaccine passports were merely an early, though significant, step for the emerging biosecurity surveillance regime. As Doug Farrow observed when commenting on vaccine passports, "We are not dealing with a [pandemic] exit strategy at all, but rather with an *entrance* strategy for the new Lords of the World."[60]

The Transhumanist Dream

Which brings us to the weird part. Meet Yuval Noah Harari, a man chock-full of big ideas. Here's a small sampling from some of his recent interviews: "Covid is critical because this is what convinces people to accept, to legitimize, total biometric surveillance. If we want to stop this epidemic, we need not just to monitor people, we need to monitor what's happening under their skin." In a recent *60 Minutes* interview with Anderson Cooper, Harari repeated this idea: "What we have seen so far is corporations and governments collecting data about where we go, who we meet, what movies we watch. The next phase is the surveillance going under our skin." He likewise told *India Today*, when commenting on changes accepted by the population during the pandemic:

We're now seeing mass surveillance systems established even in democratic countries, which previously rejected them, and we also see a change in the nature of surveillance. Previously, surveillance was mainly above the skin; now it's going under the skin. Governments want to know not just where we go or who we meet. Above all they want to know what is happening under our skin: What's our body temperature? What's our blood pressure? What is our medical condition?[61]

Harari is clearly a man who wants to . . . get under your skin. He just might succeed. Another recent interview finds him waxing philosophical: "Now humans are developing even bigger powers than ever before. We are really acquiring divine powers of creation and destruction. We are really upgrading humans into gods. We are acquiring, for instance, the power to re-engineer [human] life."[62] As Kierkegaard once said of Hegel when he talks about the Absolute, when Harari talks about the future, he sounds like he's going up in a balloon.

Another interview shows him worrying (I can't imagine why) that people are losing trust in scientific institutions: "In recent years we saw populist politicians undermining deliberately the trust that people have in important institutions like universities, like respectable media outlets. These populist politicians told people that, say, scientists are this small elite disconnected from the real people."[63] When he's not defending science against its detractors, Harari returns frequently to philosophical and theological themes, opining, for example, in his talk at Google, "I mean, all this story about Jesus rising from the dead and being the Son of God, this is fake news."[64]

Forgive me, but a few last nuggets from Professor Harari will round out the picture of his philosophy and his lofty hopes and dreams: "Humans are now hackable animals. You know, the whole idea that humans have . . . this soul or spirit and they have free will and nobody knows what's happening inside me, so, whatever I choose, whether in the election or whether in the supermarket, that's my free will—that's over."[65] Harari explains that to hack human beings you need a lot of computing power and a lot of biometric data, something not possible until recently. In a hundred years, he argues, "people could look back and identify the coronavirus epidemic as the moment "when a new regime of surveillance took over, especially surveillance under the skin, which I think is the most important development of the twenty-first century—is this ability to hack human beings."[66]

I could go on, but you get the picture. At this point you may be tempted to dismiss Harari as nothing more than an overheated, sci-fi-obsessed village atheist. After years binging on science fiction novels, the balloon of his imagination now perpetually floats up somewhere above the ether. Why should we pay any heed to this man's prognostications and prophecies?

It turns out that Harari is a professor of history at the Hebrew University of Jerusalem. His bestselling books have sold over 20 million copies worldwide, which is no small shakes. More important, he is one of the darlings of the World Economic Forum and a key architect of its agenda. In 2018 his lecture at the WEF, "Will the Future Be Human?," was sandwiched between addresses from German chancellor Angela Merkel and French president Emmanuel Macron. So he's playing in the sandbox with the big shots.

In his WEF lecture Harari explained that in the coming generations we will "learn how to engineer bodies and brains and minds," such that these will become "the main products of the twenty-first-century economy: not textiles and vehicles and weapons, but bodies and brains and minds." The few masters of the economy, he explains, will be the people who own and control data: "Today, data is the most important asset in the world," in contrast to ancient times when land was the most important asset, or the industrial age when machines were paramount.[67] WEF kingpin Klaus Schwab echoed Harari's ideas when he explained: "One of the features of the Fourth Industrial Revolution is that it doesn't change what we are doing; it changes us," through gene editing and other biotechnological tools that operate under our skin.[68]

Even the dreamy-eyed Harari admits there are some potential dangers with these developments: "If too much data is concentrated in too few hands, humanity will split not into classes but into *two different species*."[69] That would not, one supposes, be a good thing. But all things considered, he is more than willing to take these risks and forge ahead with this agenda. To be fair, Harari does not advocate for a future totalitarian state or rule by all-powerful corporations but hopes to warn us of coming dangers. In an exceptionally naïve proposal, however, Harari believes that the obvious problems posed by a tyrannical biosecurity state can be solved with *more* surveillance, by having citizens simply surveil the government: "Turn it around," he said in a talk at the Athens Democracy Forum, "Surveil the governments more. I mean, technology can always go both ways. If they can surveil us, we can surveil them."[70] This proposal is—not to put too fine a point on it—incredibly stupid. As most of us learned in kindergarten, two wrongs don't make a right.

Harari is among the more prominent members of a new species of academics, activists, and "visionaries" that refer to themselves as transhumanists. These folks aim to use technology not to alter the lived environment but to fundamentally alter human nature itself. The goal is to "upgrade" or "enhance" human beings. This is both possible and desirable, as Harari explains, because all organisms—whether humans or amoebas or bananas or viruses—are, at bottom, just "biological algorithms." Recall the eugenics ideology described in the prologue: here we have a turbocharged version of the same thing, techno-upgraded with the tools of gene editing, nanotechnology, robotics, and advanced pharmaceuticals. Transhumanism is microwaved eugenics.

The twentieth-century eugenicists referred to disabled persons as "useless eaters." Echoing this rhetoric on multiple occasions, Harari has puzzled over the question of what to do with people in the future who will refuse artificial intelligence–mediated enhancement—folks he refers to as "useless people." "The biggest question maybe in economics and politics in the coming decades," he predicts, "will be what to do with all these useless people?" He goes on to explain, "The problem is more boredom, what to do with them, and how will they find some sense of meaning in life when they are basically meaningless, worthless."[71]

Harari suggests one possible solution to the problem of what to do with useless people: "My best guess at present is a combination of drugs and computer games." Well, at least we have a head start on that, a fact that does not escape Harari's attention: "You see more and more people spending more and more time, or solving their problems with drugs and computer games, both legal drugs and illegal drugs," he explains. This is where Harari predicts those who refuse to be hacked for AI-enhancement purposes will find themselves.[72]

Encountering Harari's thought was not my first brush with the transhumanist movement. Several years ago I spoke on a panel at Stanford University sponsored by the Zephyr Institute on the topic of transhumanism. I critiqued the idea of "human enhancement," the use of biomedical technology not to heal the sick but to make the healthy "better than well," that is, bigger, faster, stronger, smarter, and so on. The event was well attended by several students from the transhumanist club at Stanford.

We had a cordial discussion, and I enjoyed chatting with these students after the talk. I learned the symbol of their student group was H+ ("humanity plus"). They were exceptionally bright, ambitious, and serious young men and women—typical Stanford students. Some of them had read their Plato in addition to their *Scientific American*. They sincerely wanted to make the world better. Perhaps there was a closet authoritarian or two among them, but my impression was that they had no interest in facilitating world domination by oligarchic corporatist regimes empowered to hack human beings.

Nevertheless, I got the impression that they did not comprehend the implications of the axioms they had accepted. We can choose our first principles, our foundational premises, but then we must follow them out to their logical conclusions; otherwise, we deceive ourselves. These students were not outliers but representative of the local culture: transhumanism is enormously influential in Silicon Valley and shapes the imagination of many of the most influential tech elites. Proponents include the Oxford University philosopher Nick Bostrom, Harvard geneticist George Church, the late physicist Stephen Hawking, engineer and inventor Ray Kurzweil, and other notables.

Returning to Harari's 2018 talk at the WEF, we hear him not only admit that control of data might enable human elites to build digital dictatorships, but also opine that hacking humans may facilitate something even more radical: "Elites may gain the power to re-engineer the future of life itself." With his Davos audience warmed up he then waxes to a crescendo: "This will be not just the greatest revolution in the history of humanity; this will be the greatest revolution in biology since the beginning of life four billion years ago." Which is, of course, a pretty big deal. Because for billions of years, nothing fundamental changed in the basic rules of the game of life, as he explains: "All of life for four billion years—dinosaurs, amoebas, tomatoes, humans—all of life was subject to the laws of natural selection and to the laws of organic biochemistry." But not anymore. As he explains, all this is about to change:

> Science is replacing evolution by natural selection with evolution by intelligent design—not the intelligent design of some god above the clouds, but our intelligent design, and the intelligent design of our clouds: the IBM Cloud, the Microsoft Cloud—these are the new driving forces of evolution. And at the same time, science may enable life—after being confined for four billion years to the limited realm of organic compounds—science may enable life to break out into the inorganic realm.[73]

The opening sentence here perfectly echoes the original definition of eugenics from the man who coined the term in the late nineteenth century, Sir Francis Galton, as quoted in the prologue: "What nature does blindly, slowly, and ruthlessly [evolution by natural selection], man may do providently, quickly, and kindly [evolution by our own—or by the cloud's—intelligent design]." But what is Harari talking about in that last sentence—life breaking out into the inorganic realm?

It's been a transhumanist dream from the dawn of modern computing that someday we will be able to upload the informational content of our brains, or our minds (if you believe in minds), into some sort of massive computing system or digital cloud or other technological repository capable of storing massive amounts of data. On this materialist view of man, we will then have no more need for our human bodies, which, after all, always fail us in the end. Shedding this mortal coil—this organic dust that always returns to dust—we will find the technological means to . . . well, *to live forever*. Living forever in the digital cloud or the mainframe computer constitutes the transhumanists' eschatology: salvation by digital technology.

This project is physically (and metaphysically) impossible, of course, because man is an inextricable unity of body and soul—not some ghost in the machine, not merely a bit of software transferable to another piece of hardware. But set that aside for now; look instead at what this eschatological dream tells us about the transhumanist movement. These imaginative flights of fancy have obviously moved well beyond the realm of science. Transhumanism is clearly a religion—a particular type of neo-Gnostic religion, as I will show at the end of this chapter. It attracts adherents today—including educated, wealthy, powerful, culturally influential adherents—because it taps into unfulfilled, deeply religious aspirations and longings.

● ● ●

I mentioned earlier the importance for our time of C. S. Lewis's book *The Abolition of Man*. Lewis once remarked that his dystopian novel *That Hideous Strength*, the third installment in his "space trilogy," was *The Abolition of Man* in fictional form. Those who have learned from Huxley's *Brave New World* and Orwell's *Nineteen Eighty-Four* would do well also to read *That Hideous Strength*, an underappreciated entry in the dystopian fiction genre. Back in 1945 Lewis foresaw Yuval Harari and his transhumanist ilk on the horizon. He brilliantly satirized their ideology in one of the novel's characters, Filostrato, an earnest but deeply misguided Italian scientist.

In the story a cabal of technocrats take over a bucolic university town in England—think of Oxford or Cambridge—and go to work immediately transforming things according to their vision of the future. The protagonist, Mark Studdock, is recruited away from the university to the technocrats' new institute. Mark desires above all to be part of the progressive set, the "inner ring" that is steering the next big thing. He spends his first several days at the N.I.C.E. (National Institute for Coordinated Experiments) trying in vain to ascertain exactly what his new job description entails. Eventually he figures out that he has been retained mainly to write propaganda explaining the institute's activities to the public. Somewhat dispirited—he is a scholar of the social sciences, after all, not a journalist—he sits down at lunch one day with Filostrato, a member of the N.I.C.E. inner circle, and learns a bit about this scientist's worldview.

It happens that Filostrato has just given orders to cut down some beech trees on the institute's property and replace them with trees made of aluminum. Someone at the table naturally asks why, remarking that he rather liked the beech trees. "Oh, yes, yes," replies Filostrato. "The pretty trees, the garden trees. But not the savages. I put the rose in my garden, but not the brier. The forest tree is a weed." Filostrato explains that he once saw a metal tree in Persia, "so natural it would deceive," which he believes could be perfected. His interlocutor objects that a tree made of metal would hardly be the same as a real tree. But the scientist is undeterred and explains why the artificial tree is superior:

> "But consider the advantages! You get tired of him in one place: two workmen carry him somewhere else: wherever you please. It never dies. No leaves to fall, no twigs, no birds building nests, no muck and mess."

"I suppose one or two, as curiosities, might be rather amusing."

"Why one or two? At present, I allow, we must have forests, for the atmosphere. Presently we find a chemical substitute. And then, why any natural trees? I foresee nothing but the art tree all over the earth. In fact, we clean the planet."

When asked if he means that there would be no vegetation at all, Filostrato replies, "Exactly. You shave your face: even, in the English fashion, you shave him every day. One day we shave the planet." Someone wonders what the birds will make of it, but Filostrato has a plan for them too: "I would not have any birds either. On the art tree I would have the art birds all singing when you press a switch inside the house. When you are tired of the singing you switch them off. Consider again the improvement. No feathers dropped about, no nests, no eggs, no dirt."

Mark replies that this sounds like abolishing pretty much all organic life. "And why not?" Filostrato counters. "It is simple hygiene." And then, echoing the rhetoric of Yuval Harari, we hear Filostrato's soaring peroration, which would have been right at home in the World Economic Forum's annual meeting in Davos:

> Listen, my friends. If you pick up some rotten thing and find this organic life crawling over it, do you not say, "Oh, the horrid thing. It is alive," and then drop it? . . . And you, especially you English, are you not hostile to any organic life except your own on your own body? Rather than permit it you have invented the daily bath. . . . And what do you call dirty dirt? Is it not precisely the organic? Minerals are clean dirt. But the real filth is what comes from organisms—sweat, spittles, excretions. Is not your whole idea of purity one huge example? The impure and the organic are interchangeable conceptions. . . . After all we are organisms ourselves.

I grant it . . . in us organic life has produced Mind. It has done its work. After that we want no more of it. We do not want the world any longer furred over with organic life, like what you call the blue mold—all sprouting and budding and breeding and decaying. We must get rid of it. By little and little, of course. Slowly we learn how. Learn to make our brains live with less and less body: learn to build our bodies directly with chemicals, no longer have to stuff them full of dead brutes and weeds. Learn how to reproduce ourselves without copulation.[74]

Someone interjects that this last part does not sound like much fun, but Filostrato responds, "My friend, you have already separated the Fun, as you call it, from fertility. The Fun itself begins to pass away. . . . Nature herself begins to throw away the anachronism. When she has thrown it away, then real civilization becomes possible."[75]

In both the real character of Harari and the fictional character of Filostrato we find men who embrace, indeed celebrate, the idea that human beings can shed the messy business of organic life and somehow transfer our bodily existence into sterile, inorganic matter. We encounter in both characters the kind of man who wants to bleach the entire earth with hand sanitizer. Were we not nudged, perhaps a bit too far, in the direction of Filostrato's dream during the pandemic, as we attempted to fully disinfect and sanitize our lived environments?

Organic matter is alive, whereas inorganic matter is dead. I can only conclude that the transhumanists' dream is, in the last analysis, a philosophy of death. But we must grant that it has become an influential philosophy among many of today's elites. In one way or another, all of us were seduced during the pandemic by the notion that by massively coordinated vigilance and the application of technology, we could rid our lived environments of pathogens and scrub our world entirely clean.

Hippocratic versus Technocratic Medicine

After that dizzying flight into the Promethean dream of the trans-humanists, our balloon can descend from Professor Harari's stratosphere back to earth, to biotechnological developments closer to home. Many of our technocrats seem undeterred by the failure of public health policies and associated new technologies to mitigate the covid pandemic. Consider, for example, Pfizer's and Moderna's mRNA vaccines. How successful was this technology in its first large-scale trial run in humans?

A useful metric to cut through a lot of statistical noise is all-cause mortality. We can argue about the causes of death—Did this person die *with* covid or *from* covid? Was this fatality a vaccine side effect or a random temporal association?—but we cannot argue about the body count. It is hard to spin death certificates. A recent preprint study in the medical journal *The Lancet* found that the mRNA vaccines showed no net benefit for all-cause mortality.[76]

Furthermore, CDC data, as well as data provided by life insurance companies stratified by age, showed a 40 percent rise in all-cause mortality among working-age adults (eighteen-to-sixty-four-year-olds) in 2021 during the mass vaccination campaign, as compared to the previous five-year baseline. To put this into context, actuaries tell us that a 10 percent rise in all-cause mortality is a once in 200-year disastrous event. The United States didn't see this kind of spike even during World War II. When age groups were further stratified, life insurance mortality in quarter three of 2021 during the mass vaccination campaign showed even more alarming excess-mortality statistics among middle-aged adults (81 percent increase for twenty-five-to-thirty-four-year-olds, 117 percent for thirty-five-to-forty-four-year-olds, 108 percent for forty-five-to-fifty-four-year-olds, and 70 percent for fifty-five-to-sixty-four-year-olds).[77]

Most of these excess deaths were not due to covid. Nor can missed screenings and medical appointments during lockdowns account for most of these deaths. If you miss a colonoscopy, you don't die the following year of colon cancer; you get a slight elevation in your risk of dying from cancer sometime in the next ten to twenty years. Likewise, if you have diabetes and miss your routine primary care appointments for a year, you might consequently have poorly controlled blood sugar for several months. This leads not to death a year later, but to a mildly elevated risk of diabetic complications much further down the road. Something else—something sudden and acute—happened in 2021 that massively affected mortality for young and middle-aged adults.

Our public health establishment has shown no interest in examining this disaster; this total disinterest is a barometer of their priorities. However, along with other concerned doctors and scientists, I've begun working with insurance industry executives and regulators who are keen on getting answers regarding vaccine safety and other potential causes of this dramatically increased mortality. But regardless of whether it turns out that vaccines caused net harm, it's at least clear that the mRNA vaccines produced no net mortality benefits for the population. (It may turn out that an age-stratified analysis will reveal overall benefit for the elderly offset by overall harm to the young—the jury is still out. My read of the current data suggests that any benefits to some populations will remain short-term and will be offset by longer-term problems.)

We were reassured time and again by the health establishment that mRNA vaccines would not alter our DNA. The conventional dogma in genetics for many years was that DNA is transcribed to RNA which is translated into proteins: the arrow moved only in this direction, or so we thought. But we now know the direction can sometimes be reversed by enzymes such as reverse transcriptase, the mechanism found in HIV viruses. A recent study found that mRNA from the covid vaccines was inserted into the DNA of human liver cells in the lab (in vitro).[78] This finding needs to be reproduced in animal models (in vivo), but this study suggests that the reassurances that these vaccines could not change our DNA may have been premature. We are learning as we go with this technology: shooting first and asking questions later.

Despite the lackluster performance of the mRNA platform in its first mass rollout, enthusiasts remain undeterred. According to advocates, this was merely an early experiment for these genetic therapies (one cannot plausibly call them vaccines any longer, even with the CDC's changing its definition of vaccine last year to accommodate these products). One notable mRNA technology enthusiast, Jamie Metzl, has an impressive pedigree. According to his bio, Metzl is "a leading technology futurist" and member of the WHO's international advisory committee on human genome editing.[79] He is the author of five books, including *Hacking Darwin: Genetic Engineering and the Future of Humanity*, a title that would no doubt excite Yuval Harari and his friends. Mr. Metzl also previously served on the U.S. National Security Council and with the United Nations.

He recently published an article in *Newsweek* on the future of mRNA technologies with the headline, "Miraculous mRNA Vaccines Are Only the Beginning." Metzl claims that these vaccines offer an "early look at how the miraculous tools of the genetics revolution will transform our health care and our world over the coming years." We now have powers to hack our DNA, he opines, and "the new vaccines are perfect early examples of this 'godlike technology.'" These are his words, not mine. Metzl explains, "The vaccines, in essence, transform our bodies into personalized manufacturing plants producing an otherwise foreign object to trigger our natural immune response."

The possibilities are endless, he waxes: "This approach will soon create a whole new platform for fighting cancers and other diseases, as well as for providing enhancements even more profound than vaccination." While these transformations were well underway before the pandemic, covid "supercharged the genetics revolution," which "will soon touch our lives ever more intimately." This revolution will include not just enormous advances in agriculture, industry, and medicine, it will also "recast our evolutionary trajectory as a species."[80] As bioethicist Leon Kass once summarized the gene-editing project, "human nature now lies on the operating table."[81]

Metzl acknowledges there are some risks: he specifically mentions the possibility of crashing entire ecosystems, engaging in unethical and dangerous human experimentation, fostering discriminatory practices, exacerbating inequalities, and engineering our own undoing. But like Harari he believes these risks are worth taking to gain the potential payoffs: "Awareness of these risks should not prevent us from charging forward," as he puts it. Perhaps charging forward is an inapposite verb, but Mr. Metzl, a WHO advisor on gene editing, is nothing if not enthusiastic about this agenda.

To his credit—and here I agree with him—he advises, "The future of our species and world is too important to be left to a small number of experts and officials. We each need to take responsibility for educating ourselves on these critical issues. . . . We must all be informed, empowered citizens demanding accountability from our leaders at all levels."[82] These are, indeed, among the reasons I wrote this book. It's not clear, however, how Mr. Metzl believes a process of democratic input will shape the use of genetic technologies.

A full exploration of the ethics of gene editing lies outside the scope of this book. For now, I want to briefly examine mRNA vaccines as a window into fundamental questions informing our use of biotechnology. This discussion will help us better understand some philosophical presuppositions undergirding the biomedical security state. I am indebted to Stefano Zamagni, a brilliant young scholar I shared a panel with last year, for some of his insights here, which spurred my own thinking about mRNA vaccines and similar genetic technologies.

Covid was the first pandemic of the technological age, the age of the triumph of science. With the arrival of this pathogen, we were suddenly confronted with something that we could not control. This was an especially terrifying prospect for people who have grown used to the idea that we have already achieved technological mastery over the vicissitudes of nature. This notion of asserting technical control over the wild expanse of nature is deeply embedded in the American psyche, as suggested by the idea of manifest destiny. Pragmatism is the default American philosophy—insofar as we have a public philosophy—and pragmatism ratifies the worship of force, the cult of industrial power over the natural world.[83]

Some pandemic observers in 2020 opined that covid represented the defeat, or at least the demotion, of our scientific and technological pretentions. The hubris of scientism appeared to be knocked down several notches by the new virus. Many people assumed that covid would force us to recognize that we are not in complete control of nature but remain fragile and dependent. But Zamagni argues the opposite:

> The decision to impose a general lockdown is not an indication of the defeat of science, but entirely to the contrary. It shines a light on the common presupposition that, confronted with any serious issue, only science can possibly offer a way forward. When science was (temporarily) in difficulty, there simply could be no other possibility but to stop all of public life and wait for scientific and technological development to take its course, offering the necessary conditions for a return to life. The lockdown, which was then followed by the vaccine, marks, then, the victory of a scientistic and pragmatic [philosophical] anthropology according to which man's life is determined by his ability to adapt to ever new conditions through ever-new inventions.[84]

Science had temporarily met its match with covid, but our implicit worship of technological power continued undeterred. The ideology of scientism soldiered on, shaping our entire response to the pandemic: As Zamagni explains, "Scientism and technocracy constitute the ocean in which we swim, so much so that the possibility of framing human existence in any other way hardly comes to mind." He goes on to say that, in the spirit of technocratic pragmatism, "disease and death, which humanity has to deal with in a special way during a time of epidemic, are conceived as 'problems to be solved,' instead of 'realities to be faced.'"[85] The commitment to lockdowns and forced mass vaccination as the only feasible solution to the pandemic was from the outset ideological, not scientific. The scientific evidence now shows this plan to have been a failure in terms of pandemic management. But we continue to cling to the same illusions that drove this strategy.

Traditional Hippocratic medicine sees the human body as the primary agent of health and healing. The body is an integrated, organic whole, naturally oriented to health and human flourishing. However, the body encounters threats and obstacles to the realization of these ends in the form of disease and injury. Medicine's primary role is to remove these obstacles so that the body can heal itself. A surgeon does not really "close" a surgical wound; she merely positions the tissues together with sutures so that the body can heal the wound. Since it is naturally oriented toward health and wholeness, the body does most of the work.

Similarly, antibiotics alone do not rid the body of infections; they merely lower the infectious load sufficiently to allow the body's own immune system to eradicate the pathogen. For this reason, antibiotics are of no avail in a patient who is too severely immunocompromised, as happens in advanced AIDS, for example. Again, in this example, the body is the primary agent of healing. Good medicine works with the body as its assistant, in a subordinate role. Nature is the norm of health for Hippocratic medicine.

By introducing part of a virus, or an inactivated virus that cannot infect and replicate, a traditional vaccine works by stimulating the immune system to produce an immune response to the modified pathogen. This permits the body to eradicate the pathogen more effectively when it encounters the real thing. Sound medicine requires us to rigorously examine the safety and efficacy of any specific vaccine, of course. But as a general principle, the traditional vaccines aim to help the body mimic, to the greatest extent possible, natural infection-induced immunity, albeit without making the person sick. In this model, the body in its normal functioning remains the primary agent of healing, spurred along by the vaccine. The medical intervention facilitates and extends the body's own immune system, without treating the body as dumb matter to be entirely externally manipulated.

The mRNA vaccines differ in fundamental ways, arguably departing from this Hippocratic paradigm. Zamagni maintains that "this particular vaccine more than others is a technological device, and thus it enshrines a technocratic understanding of the human being."[86] Here's what he means: unlike traditional vaccines, the mRNA therapeutics utilize a command-and-control mechanism, hijacking our cellular biology and redirecting our body's "machinery" for novel purposes—in this case, the production of the virus's spike protein, which is then expressed on our own cells. This process has nothing whatsoever to do with the natural workings of a healthy human body.

Whatever therapeutic effect the mRNA vaccines were supposed to achieve, they did so by "acting upon the body in a violent and manipulative way," in Zamagni's description. This technological device's relationship to the body is one of *power*, not one of *assistance*. The mRNA technology does not facilitate the body's natural ends or intrinsic purposes, as traditional vaccines arguably do. The mRNA device instrumentalizes the body, whose functioning and purpose is imposed from the outside. The body's innate immune function is not assisted and facilitated, but "deeply modified in its essence," as our cellular machinery is manipulated extrinsically by this technology.

Zamagni explains some of the implications of this shift, which include the necessary exclusion of natural immunity as a legitimate category:

> It is not the [mRNA] vaccine that depends on the human body, in which case it could be defined as an "immunizing instrument" insofar as it is the extension of the body's "self-immunizing" capacity. On the contrary, the acquisition of natural immunity is bracketed out and even totally neglected, so that the body is made (mechanically) dependent on the vaccine and defined as *per se* non-working and working only if and as "vaccinated." Note that the political debate, in the U.S. at least, tends to ignore that there are millions of people who have "naturally acquired immunity." Only the vaccines are admitted as "therapeutic."[87]

In arguing for the recognition of natural immunity in our public health policies, my lawsuit against the University of California is not just challenging sloppy interpretations of science, it is also challenging a degraded philosophy of medicine. The mRNA vaccination program, with its calls for frequent boosters as vaccine efficacy rapidly wanes, suggests a mechanistic view of human beings as mere hardware that requires software updates two or three times a year to remain functional. Indeed, it is no accident that this technology is pushed by people like Bill Gates, who literally think that biological viruses are like computer viruses which can be stopped with the right antivirus mRNA "software." Overzealous computer geeks seem not to realize that "computer virus" is merely a loose metaphor, and that the two types of viruses—digital and biological—are nothing alike.

In the mechanistic-technocratic ideology of scientism, *there is no such thing as human nature*, defined by the proper functioning of an organic body with its own intrinsic ends. The body is reduced to dumb matter, inert raw material that might just as well be dead as alive. The transhumanists can at least be given credit for drawing out the logical conclusions of this philosophy of life: the body can eventually be discarded in favor of cleaner and less messy inorganic substrates for human consciousness.

For the technocratic mindset, the reference point for medicine is no longer the healthy human body as an integrated whole, which needs to be supported and maintained by working with the body's own innate capacities. The reference point for medicine is literally the corpse—or at least the sick body—which needs to be technologically vivified and periodically updated from the outside. On this conception, the human body has no form in itself: it is merely a grab bag of discreet physiological functions, each of which can be externally commandeered and reconfigured.

It's no wonder, then, that today's technocrats believe we should "hack" the body so that we can impose upon it whichever form we wish. On this view, the body's physiological hardware can do whatever our engineered software tells it to do. We can theoretically program the entire operating code for the body from start to finish. The human body, and thus the human person, is no longer a subject but an object, mere raw material for external manipulation. Man's unique subjectivity, his interiority, disappears. In Del Noce's striking formulation, "The characteristic perfectibility of the world of technology constantly perfects depersonalization."[88]

This has profound consequences for human self-understanding. Consider, for example, just one of the reversals of our assumptions during the pandemic. People used to be presumed healthy until proven sick: you needed a doctor's note if you missed too many days of work. But during the pandemic people were assumed to be sick until proven healthy: you needed ubiquitous and never-ending asymptomatic testing to allow you to work, travel, gather, and so on. Or your immune system was assumed to be subfunctional until you downloaded the latest mRNA software update in the form of a jab.

Ghosts in the Machine

The scientistic-technocratic assumptions about health and the human body undergirding mRNA interventions are consonant with transhumanist views of humanity. The latter promises that we will eliminate not only disease but also human suffering and hardship, if only we fully embrace the new genetic interventions and their promise of limitless self-determination. As I already suggested, transhumanism is not just a view of science and its uses, but a religion—one that promises salvation not vertically in eternity but horizontally in the future. It is, in fact, a particular type of religion: a technologically updated version of ancient Gnostic religions.

Gnosticism was a form of religious thought that constituted the Church's main competitor in the early centuries of Christianity. The various Gnostic religious sects that proliferated in antiquity shared a common disdain for the material world, including the human body.

Notwithstanding its ascetical tendencies, rooted in the doctrine of Christ's salvific suffering on the cross, Christianity could despise neither the material world nor the human body: the doctrines of creation and the incarnation were bulwarks against that option.

For the Gnostics, by contrast, only the spiritual realm was good and created by a good God; they saw the material world as the creation of an evil principle. The lawfully ordered material world, the world studied by the natural sciences, was an obstacle to human liberation. The essential element of all Gnostic thought was rebellion against the idea of a cosmic order inscribed in material reality, as Del Noce explained:

> The Gnostics do not deny to the world the attribute of order, but they interpret it as an abomination rather than a good. They do not say that the cosmos is disordered, but that it is governed by a rigid and hostile order, by a tyrannical and cruel law. Their God is not just outside and beyond the world, but against the world, and this is where they break away from Christianity. Moral rebellion reflects a metaphysical rebellion. Therefore, the Gnostic position leads to the obliteration of ethics, as refusal to respect being and to be faithful to objective norms. This refusal was the common root of two opposite attitudes [found among the ancient Gnostics], libertinism as desecration of reality and asceticism as its radical rejection.[89]

The last sentence refers to the two tendencies found among the various Gnostic sects in terms of their treatment of the human body: some took the path of extreme asceticism in matters of food, drink, and sex—the path of rejecting the body and its capacities. Others became extreme libertines in these matters—the path of desecration of the body. Although these extremes appear at first glance to be opposed, both tendencies evince the same underlying disdain for the body as an ordered, organic whole oriented toward human flourishing. Extreme asceticism and extreme libertinism both treat the body instrumentally, rather than as a constitutive part of the human person. For the Gnostics, we are not ensouled bodies but ghosts in the machine. And the machine—the human body—is dispensable.

If material creation is the work of a principle hostile to human liberation, as the Gnostics believed, the notion of man's being in the image and likeness of God makes no sense. Wholesale rejection and desecration, total rebellion against the established order, are justified in the name of liberating humanity from this inherently oppressive world. This rebellion requires a type of violence capable of rupturing the continuum of history. Recall the language of disruption and historical discontinuity found among both totalitarians and transhumanists. The future does not involve the fulfillment of the past but rather its total negation, as we saw in the totalitarianisms of the previous century. A wholly new age is nigh, the transhumanist clerics likewise preach, with changes not seen since the origins of life four billion years ago.

While Christianity proclaimed that salvation is in principle offered to everyone regardless of status or ability, Gnosticism posited that only a few select elites could be initiated into the deep mysteries, and thus only a few are privy to the deepest truths about the world. Today's neo-Gnostic clerisy likewise assumes that only the elites are fully awake to the direction of history; only they are sufficiently enlightened to steer the masses. In the classical Platonic view, affirmed also by the early Christian apologists, right and wrong are, in principle, knowable to all human beings through their conscience. The light of conscience participates in a universally shared rationality: this is our point of contact with the *logos* that orders the cosmos and draws us toward the good. This Platonic doctrine continued in various forms through ancient, medieval, and key strands of modern philosophy—from Aristotle and Plotinus among the ancients to Rosmini and Scheler in the nineteenth and twentieth centuries.

In the Gnostic view, by contrast, the direction of history, which is the source of ethics, cannot be the object of rational persuasion. This outlook inevitably separates a class of political and intellectual elites from the unenlightened masses. The initiated Gnostics have special insight into the direction of history, whereas the crowds can only be swayed by propaganda. After all, appealing to the rationality of the masses makes no sense when language and reason are purely instrumental, rather than a common inheritance, as we saw in the first chapter. The propaganda deployed by elites might make use of traditional moral terms—such as goodness, justice, peace, democracy, solidarity, and so forth—but such words are, at bottom, meaningless. Language is a tool of power, not a means for communicating truth. The falsification of language is baked into the system. Newspeak is necessary.

Del Noce saw that the ancient Gnostic religions resurfaced in the twentieth century by claiming to be "scientific." Pure nihilistic atheism is very difficult for most people to live, so they tend to seek substitutes in various neo-Gnostic religions. Scientism and its associated technocratic worldview represent this old religious system clothed in new technological garb. Other contemporary trends—from the New Age movement to gender theory—are similarly Gnostic in their essence. Today's transhumanist neo-Gnostics, like their ancient counterparts, believe that escape from this oppressive material order is possible with the full use of one's own technological powers, deployed to fundamentally recreate oneself. The goal is a radical rejection of any form of dependence in favor of radically new forms of self-creation.

But technologically mediated liberation from the constraints and givens of embodied human existence may not turn out to be so liberating. Early experiments in this program over the last several years suggest that this vision may be an illusion, perhaps eventually a dystopian nightmare. Long experience has shown that the Hippocratic paradigm for medicine and biotechnology is humanizing and conducive to health and human flourishing. Recent experience during the pandemic suggests that the technocratic paradigm—grounded in mechanistic scientism and leading to neo-Gnostic utopian dreams—is profoundly dehumanizing.

It should be clear that the biomedical security state finds its home in the technocratic, not the Hippocratic, paradigm for medicine and biotechnology. During the pandemic, we forgot all about Hippocrates and his oath. The dream of a sanitized and deathless society that we embraced during covid "created a world where the home is a prison and friends and family are a health hazard," in the words of writer Alex Gutentag. "In this world children are told they are killing their grandparents simply by existing." She rightly worries that "we have a limited window of time to reclaim the things that make life worth living: family, community, cultural heritage, the social sphere, public institutions, common spaces, and free movement."[90]

In his important recent study *The Psychology of Totalitarianism*, Mattias Desmet shows that totalitarian societies always try to replace nature with a rationally controlled artificial system. As we have seen, this is precisely what the technocratic paradigm for biotechnology does to the human body. And as I argued in the opening chapter, the scientism that undergirds this paradigm is intrinsically totalitarian. The rising biomedical security state—with its mass surveillance, its temporary licenses to live, its contingent vouchers to buy and sell, and its coercive medical mandates—a system in which dissidents are punished through exclusion, has already shown itself to contain the seeds of new forms of totalitarianism.

With virtually no pushback, we have already allowed many unjust and harmful measures to advance. Our general goodwill and civic-mindedness were nullified by misplaced trust and self-protective timidity. During covid, cowardice often masqueraded as civility. It is not too late, neither is it too early, to change course and mount firm resistance. It's time to heed the great Soviet dissident, Aleksandr Solzhenitsyn, who wrote in *The Gulag Archipelago*, "If . . . If . . . If only we had stood together against the common threat, we could easily have defeated it. So, why didn't we? . . . We didn't love freedom enough. And even more—we had no awareness of the real situation. . . . We hurried to submit. We submitted with pleasure! We purely and simply deserved everything that happened afterward."[91]

The hour is later than we may think. Twilight is near. Continued compliance with manifestly unjust and often absurd mandates and arbitrary strictures, whether now or in the next declared crisis, will not return us to a normal functioning society. Since the pandemic began, every good-faith or selfless act of compliance on the part of citizens only resulted in more illogical pandemic "countermeasures" that further eroded our civil liberties, harmed our overall health, and undermined human flourishing.

There is a human right not enshrined in any constitution: the right to the truth. No right has been more systematically trammeled over the last three years. Why, I ask, did our public health authorities acknowledge certain truths only after the damage from the lies had already been done—only, for example, after tens of thousands lost their jobs due to coercive mandates that did nothing to advance public health? Who will hold our leaders accountable for this?

Regarding future medical mandates and other coercive measures: nonviolent resistance and civil disobedience constitute the right and just path forward. I maintain that firm resistance to the point of civil disobedience is not only permissible under the circumstances, but required if we are to prevent this twilight from fading into night.

CHAPTER 4

Reclaiming Freedom: Human Flourishing in a More Rooted Future

Until they become conscious they will never rebel, and until after they have rebelled they cannot become conscious.

—*George Orwell*, Nineteen Eighty-Four

We can now summarize the central features of The New Abnormal. The rising biomedical security state . . .

1. Begins with the militarization of public health, leading to the melding of public health with the police powers of the state, facilitated by digital technologies of surveillance and control. Within this framework, real, known, present human goods are sacrificed on the altar of theoretical, unknown, future biological risks.

2. Dictates that various problems—social, environmental, economic, et cetera—be reframed as public health issues, and eventually declared public health crises. This model of governance entails jumping from one declared crisis to the next, each time invoking the need for extra-legislative or extra-judicial executive powers to manage the declared emergency.

3. Assumes the legal form of the state of exception triggered by ongoing emergencies: hypothetical risks according to "worst case" logic are then used to justify extreme responses requiring systematic control of the entire body of citizens. The purported protection of public health overrules any individual or privacy rights, and health is imposed on citizens as a legal obligation.

4. Drives industry toward systems of algorithmically controlled automation where humans progressively become superfluous. The human person is reduced to bare biological life—a mere collection of muscles, tendons, ligaments, and bones—with regrettable energy and excretion requirements.

5. Regards all rationality as purely instrumental, thus destroying the possibility of shared universal truths. Philosophically, its epistemology is scientism; its metaphysics is materialism; and its ethics is the direction of history as discerned by an elite clerisy.

6. Takes the religious form of revolutionary neo-Gnosticism, which seeks to overcome all embodied, material limitations. An elite class of unelected but credentialed bureaucratic managers administer the system. These technocrats move in the virtual world of screens and software while controlling the bodies of those moving in the real world of physical labor.

7. Takes the political form of corporatism, which coincides with fascism according to its original and precise meaning. This political system pushes depersonalization and alienation to the extreme, constituting a dehumanizing regime that inevitably moves toward totalitarianism.

I realize that by now our narrative may have induced in the reader a degree of pessimism. But we should take heart that the emerging biomedical security state has not advanced entirely unopposed. There have been hopeful signs of resistance, though we certainly need more.

The past year witnessed the largest mass protest movement in world history. The medical freedom movement spanned from America to Europe to Indonesia and Australia. You would be forgiven for not noticing it, since there was a near-total media blackout. However, it was hard to hide the photos and videos shared on social media, so the information is available.[1] People around the world rose up by the hundreds of thousands to demand their freedom in opposition to The New Abnormal.

The movement started in Italy in November 2021 with huge crowds gathered in Rome. Protests spread from there across the European continent, with large gatherings in the Czech Republic on November 13, Vienna on December 10, Barcelona on December 13, and Paris in the days preceding Christmas. Meanwhile, down under in Australia—which had some of the most repressive biomedical security measures in the world—huge gatherings arose in multiple cities starting in November and continued for many weeks.

Germans protested medical segregation, Parisians demanded *liberté*, and Londoners opposed vaccine mandates and other restrictions during the omicron wave. Demonstrators in Barcelona chanted for an end to mandates and totalitarianism. Italians stood up in Turin and New Zealanders resisted their autocratic prime minister who seemed intoxicated with pandemic powers, while citizens of Austria took to the streets for an entire weekend of protesting. Other mass protests were seen in unexpected places like Tbilisi, Georgia.

The Italian government had imposed a "no jab, no job" mandate on all workers in October 2021. At that time, 40 percent of the dockworkers at Italy's most important commercial port, Trieste, remained unvaccinated. Most of them refused to comply and launched an anti-mandate strike that lasted for weeks. Local police eventually removed the striking workers from the port by force. The workers then moved their protest to the main town square in Trieste. Again, the authorities removed them by force. By the end of October, the local government had banned all protests in the town's main square on the flimsy pretext of health security, that is, the worry that demonstrations might lead to covid spread.[2]

Resistance movements elsewhere often met with more forceful retaliation and repression. The biosecurity state cracked down violently on many protestors. In the Netherlands a Dutch man was roughed up by the police while being forcibly arrested for not having a vaccine passport in an outdoor Christmas market. Austrian police rounded up and arrested anti-mandate protestors, as did Canadian Mounties. Police in Belgium showed their authoritarian instincts against anti-mandate demonstrators by marching toward them in riot gear while spraying protestors with firehoses. Videos of Belgian police, later scrubbed from the internet, also showed them beating defenseless protestors. Closer to home, the NYPD arrested ten anti-mandate protestors in New York City, including their leaders, over two consecutive nights. Their crime? Sitting in two restaurants in Queens without proof of vaccination and refusing to leave. Meanwhile, apologists in the Western media gave us headlines like: "Only Surveillance Can Save Us from Coronavirus," with the lede, "Big data offers tools to stop the pandemic—if only we change our definition of privacy."[3]

We can take heart from this mass movement and its courageous participants. If you don't want the future that our biomedical security state portends, you are not alone. The resistance battle will be prolonged and arduous. Our new paradigm of governance will require ongoing crises triggering perpetual states of emergencies. When covid has exhausted all its possibilities and is no longer plausible to the masses, the next declared crisis—whether real or manufactured—will not be long in coming. Our present reprieve from the worst of the pandemic strictures will not last forever.

Among the tangible signs of hope, we should recall the impact of the Canadian truckers' Freedom Convoy, which we encountered in the opening of this book's first chapter. Following the Trudeau government's brutal crackdown on the weeks-long Freedom Convoy demonstration in

Ottawa, other pro-freedom protests spread across Canada—with new protests emerging in February 2022 in Calgary, Toronto, Vancouver, and elsewhere across the country. Protestors in downtown Toronto held signs that read "Freedom Over Fear" and "Stop Power Abuse" as the demonstrators sang the national anthem.[4]

These courageous Canadians were aware of the risks: they had seen the widespread video footage showing police violence against the Freedom Convoy in Ottawa. Besides the use of tear gas and pepper spray, an elderly woman identified as an Indigenous elder was reportedly injured after mounted police rode through a crowd of convoy supporters.[5] Baton-wielding police officers were caught on video beating protestors and a reporter who was targeted for filming the demonstration.[6] As the truckers were forced to drive their rigs out of Ottawa, remaining protestors fist-bumped and shook their hands. A man shouted to one of one of the departing truck drivers, "You are a hero!"

Although the Ottawa gathering was forcibly dispersed, the convoy and its supporters across Canada did not back down. While Trudeau opted for intransigent force rather than alter his mandates or even negotiate with the convoy leadership, the movement won notable victories. Five Canadian provinces—Ontario, Alberta, Saskatchewan, Quebec, and Prince Edward Island—dropped their vaccine mandates during the protests, with Alberta also dropping its school mask requirement. At the national level, the Canadian government relaxed its border pandemic restrictions, which were the initial source of the truckers' complaints.

Leading politicians in Canada, including some from Trudeau's own party who broke ranks, began speaking out against mandates and expressing sympathy for the concerns expressed by the demonstrators. The public policy tide turned in Canada even as police disbanded the Ottawa protest, and public sympathy grew despite the media's slanderous attacks against the convoy. A February 2022 poll showed nearly half of Canadians said they "may not agree with everything the people who have taken part in the truck protests in Ottawa have said, but their frustration is legitimate and worthy of our sympathy."[7]

Reuters reported during the protests, "Justin Trudeau's support of vaccine mandates in fighting COVID-19 helped him win re-election five months ago, but now he looks increasingly isolated as restrictions are being lifted around the world."[8] This was reflected in the polls, as this report noted: "The Trudeau government's approval rating fell six percentage points between January 12, before the protests began, and February 8, while they were ongoing." Trudeau had condescendingly dismissed the truckers as "a small fringe minority" with "unacceptable views." But this small fringe minority managed to knock down the prime minister's approval rating and achieve many of their political aims.

We can take another lesson from the truckers: they were unfailingly cheerful and peaceful, not dire prophets of doom and gloom. As one reporter from Ottawa wrote, "There's an easy-going, happy-warrior feeling to it; music emanates from speakers in different encampments, free food and coffee is served out of makeshift booths, and truckers pray the Lord's Prayer—in English and French—every evening at 7 p.m."[9] While a few offshoots in other parts of the country were rightly criticized for occasionally blockading trade routes, for the most part, the Freedom Convoy movement was remarkably peaceful, particularly considering its decentralized, spontaneous character. With enormous political, economic, media, and finally militarized police forces arrayed against them, this grassroots, working-class mass movement succeeded in achieving key public policy victories. It also inspired similar movements elsewhere, including in the United States. We should take heart from this: ordinary people, acting together with clear objectives, are not powerless.

Nor are we yet politically impotent. Help often comes from unexpected places, and history is full of surprises and unexpected plot twists. Recent news from the May 2022 WHO meeting suggests the pandemic treaty, which appeared to be an unstoppable juggernaut, is hitting roadblocks. The Biden administration's proposed changes to the International Health Regulations met significant resistance. Opposition was coordinated by, of all places, Botswana, which led a coalition of African countries and other concerned nations. Official delegates from developed nations, including Australia, the United Kingdom, the European Union, and the United States, spoke in strong support of the amendments and urged other states to join them. But they have not succeeded in persuading Brazil, Brunei, Namibia, Bangladesh, Russia, India, China, South Africa, and Iran to embrace this tool of the West's biomedical neocolonialism. Brazil indicated it would abandon the WHO entirely rather than subject its people to these amendments. While this fight is far from over, the proposed IHR changes, at least for now, have been tabled for a future meeting.[10]

Here in the closing chapter, I hope to offer some suggestions for the medical-freedom resistance movement as we construct a better future than the one offered by the biomedical security state and its corporatist allies. No doubt wiser minds than mine will offer more creative and effective means of resistance, renewal, and policy reform. Human beings are incredibly resilient. Despite the immense challenges, I have hope for the future. Before I present some policy proposals, we need to begin with what I consider the necessary precondition for any meaningful renewal or reform.

The Sickness unto Death

The first and most necessary step is to overcome our fear. For fear, as Heidegger noted, "bewilders us and makes us 'lose our heads.'"[11] Incapacitated by fear in 2020, we discarded clear scientific information from credible authorities and instead uncritically swallowed incredible claims presented with little pretense to scientific rigor. As a psychiatrist with years of clinical experience treating patients who are paralyzed by anxiety, I can say confidently: we cannot reason clearly or act well when we are afraid. It is not by chance that we find the crystalline admonishment "be not afraid" repeated more than a hundred times in the Bible.

This includes even—and especially—the fear of death. Socrates famously claimed that all philosophy—literally, the "love of wisdom," *philo-sophia*—is a preparation for death. His own love of wisdom manifested most clearly not in his words but in his martyrdom at the hands of the Athenian democracy, the members of which could not abide his constant probing questions—questions that often undermined the establishment's pretentions. In his essay "Through Philosophy We Learn How to Die," Montaigne reminded us: "It is not certain where death awaits us, so let us await it everywhere. To think of death beforehand is to think of our liberty. Whoever learns how to die has learned how not to be a slave. Knowing how to die frees us from all subjection and constraint."[12]

Fear induces impotence, powerlessness, paralysis. It leads to withdrawal and disengagement. Fear causes separation and isolation, which prevents meaningful engagement and social solidarity. In a state of chronic fear, we can do nothing to construct a more human future. We must find the spiritual resources to overcome our fear. Only then will we regain a basic openness to the world, to reality as it stands before us.

We must also regain our historical memory, our broader perspective. Pandemics and viruses have always been, and will always be, with us. We can care for one another through these difficulties, but we need not cower in fear or give into despair. Human existence is inescapably contingent: that beautiful tree may fall upon me; that radiant sun may burn me; that limpid water may drown me or may flood my home; my fellow man may strike me or even kill me. All the same, I need not live in fear. I need not close myself off from the world and from my neighbor. We can endure hardship, we can suffer, without crumpling and without turning against one another. The enemy is not pain or illness. The enemy is fear. The enemy is hatred or indifference toward our fellow human beings.

Political power and sovereignty should never be grounded in fear, contrary to Thomas Hobbes's influential theory of the social contract. Human beings are intrinsically social animals; we are hardwired to connect. Our political life originates in this basic fact of human sociality. Our life together does not begin in some original state of nature as atomized individuals whose life is "solitary, poor nasty, brutish, and short"—a nightmare world that requires a Leviathan to guarantee our security. Our political life originates not as a reaction to external threats, but as one grounded in the fact that we are connected to one another from the beginning, made to live together in community. The bonds of family and social connection are literally inscribed in our body: just look at your belly button. Security is good, but it cannot be the highest good. And it is not the original and primary aim of the state.

As a psychiatric physician, I dive into people's pain and anguish every day. I personally suffered a severe and debilitating chronic pain condition for more than four years, spending most of those years lying on my back.[13] On one occasion the pain was so severe that I blacked out for twenty minutes. I understand the immense value of health for a flourishing human life. But even health is not our highest good, not our salvation. A life free of disease does not necessarily constitute a flourishing human life; neither does a life with disease or disability constitute a worthless existence.

The authorities that presently govern us somehow came to believe that the biomedical security state (and its associated climate of fear) was our best option in the face of a novel pathogen. I submit that they were dead wrong. Human life is fragile, to be sure, but we are not so brittle as to be unable to face new challenges with courage and clear-sightedness.

There is, I admit, a grain of truth to "the new normal" proposal: the world before the pandemic was profoundly unjust and perhaps unsustainable. We will not go back to exactly the way things were before, for history does not work that way. We look to the past not to recover a lost golden age, which never really existed, but to discern traces in time of enduring principles that can be applied in new ways to our unique present circumstances. What we need to recover is not the past, but the eternal—those perennially relevant values and principles that must find new forms of expression in every period of history.

While we might not return to the old normal, The New Abnormal—the future that our technocratic elites are rapidly putting in place—will be far more unjust and dehumanizing than the injustices of the pre-pandemic past.

It is this proposed future, conceived during the last few decades and launched during the pandemic, that we cannot accept. Whatever comes next—and none of us can foresee precisely what will follow the dissolution of the old bourgeois democracies of the West—we cannot allow it to be the vision imagined by the new lords of the world and their transhumanist clerics.

In the opening chapter, I described the biomedical security state in terms of what Lewis Mumford called, over a half-century ago, the megamachine—a machine made of human parts. He concludes his classic work with this advice: "For those of us who have thrown off the myth of the machine, the next move is ours: for the gates of the technocratic prison will open automatically, despite their rusty ancient hinges, as soon as we choose to walk out."[14] Let us begin now, without fear, to push open those doors and let in the sun.

As a practical first step, whenever you catch yourself self-censoring, try to stop. As we have seen, classical dictatorships differ from totalitarian systems; the two are not identical. Dictatorships are maintained because *people fear the sovereign*: they fear external punishments. Totalitarian systems are maintained because *people internalize the ideology*: they learn to embrace the system. Under a dictatorship the chains are external; in a totalitarian regime the chains are internal. Totalitarian systems eventually stop needing so many external censors because people internalize the interdicts and begin to censor themselves. After sufficient time, the helpless denizens of totalitarian societies don't need to bite their tongues or consciously watch what they say, for they have become incapable of having dissenting ideas.

This constitutes perhaps the worst form of slavery, an interior prison where we no longer see the prison bars. When we allow ourselves to self-censor, to stop saying what we think, to avoid raising inconvenient questions, we begin constructing that interior prison, one brick at a time. "The specific character of despair is this," Kierkegaard wrote in *The Sickness unto Death*, "it is unaware of being despair."[15]

Till We Have Faces

During the pandemic I generally steered clear of the mask wars. I saw lockdowns and vaccine mandates as more serious problems to focus my attention upon. The science on masks was clear from the outset. Prior to covid, there was not a single rigorous study showing that cloth or surgical masks, or indeed any masks outside a hospital setting, are useful for slowing the spread of respiratory viruses. The CDC initially acknowledged this, then flipped its recommendations in favor of masks. A few sloppy backfilled studies, using abstract models or highly contrived situations like mannequins wearing masks, were published to justify that recommendation. These half-hearted attempts to reinforce mask policies lacked clinical outcomes, control groups, and rigorous study methodology.

Every one of the fifteen randomized controlled trials—the gold standard of medical research—done prior to the pandemic for masks and respiratory viruses found no benefit; but somehow, we pretended these rigorous studies no longer mattered. It was long known that masks did not work for source control (preventing spread from the mask wearer to others),[16] but this notion was nevertheless seized upon as a talking point to frame masks as a social duty rather than a personal choice. The pre-pandemic public health guidelines for respiratory viruses said masks don't work. The WHO studies prior to covid found masks don't work. The high-quality studies on masks that emerged during the pandemic confirmed that masks don't work, which should not have surprised anyone familiar with the scientific literature on masks.

We were told for months that SARS-CoV-2 spreads by respiratory droplets, which surgical masks might theoretically stop. I recall hearing this falsehood repeated time and again in townhall meetings by infectious disease specialists at UCI. Before long it became clear that, on the contrary, this virus was aerosolized, not spread by droplets. Anyone who wears glasses knows they constantly fog up with a surgical or cloth mask, which means that an aerosolized virus is clearly not limited by a mask. This was confirmed by large trials that showed no benefits for clinical covid outcomes between masked and unmasked settings and regions, as well as studies documenting the collateral medical, psychological, and social harms of masks, particularly for children.[17]

Mask mandates continued, nevertheless. I found them annoying but did not focus my energies there, reasoning that vaccine mandates were far more unethical and potentially harmful. I now believe, however, that mask mandates also inflicted harms that should not be trivialized. I anticipate in the coming years we will see a growing body of research on child development, adding to the already available studies, showing how masks impede cognitive, emotional, and verbal development, likely compromising early attachment relationships and probably increasing anxiety disorders. These studies are already appearing, and the early results are concerning.

I recently returned from my first flight since the federal government lifted its mask mandate on airplanes, only to see in the paper the next morning that several universities—including Georgetown, Columbia, Johns Hopkins, and Rice—were reinstating mask mandates on campus, mandates that were phased out not long ago. College administrators, that dogged gang of clueless do-gooders, continue to obsessively track "cases," that is, positive tests irrespective of symptoms—tracking hospitalizations or deaths on campus would yield little of concern—and so the mask mania continues unabated and undeterred by evidence.

During the pandemic, masks became a kind of talisman of security, a charmed amulet to ward off infection. The psychology of this is not difficult to understand. At the start of covid, we were bombarded with terrifying news of an invisible and unknown pathogen that was killing people across the globe. This was amplified by the myth of asymptomatic spread—which made every other person a potential threat to my existence—another key element in our adoption of the biosecurity paradigm.[18] People understandably felt helpless and frightened.

Masks gave people something tangible they could do to feel less powerless and a bit more protected—whether masks in fact helped control viral transmission or not. Public health officials understood this psychological effect: when they occasionally let their own "mask" slip, several of them admitted that this was the real reason to require masks, even if their efficacy was nil—at least it gave frightened people some sense of control. If I don my mask and you don yours, I feel safer. When I dutifully put on a mask, I feel that I have exercised a little bit of agency, which reduces my distress.

Then, in a process of classical behavioral conditioning, this routine act, done to reduce one's anxiety, was reinforced many times daily for several years. It's little wonder that when talk of dropping masks surfaced, many remarked that they would *never again* feel safe at a restaurant or theater without a mask. Scores of people had great difficulty relinquishing masks, even when most mask mandates were abandoned in 2022. One young patient of mine indicated she would continue wearing a mask even after her school dropped the requirement: she admitted it was not because she was afraid of covid, but rather because she was afraid of showing her face.

Although masks were deployed (whether knowingly or unknowingly) to help people manage their fear, this psychological Band-Aid only worsened their fear in the end. Those who tried to protect themselves by wearing a mask or sheltering in place were not reassured over the long term, but only repeatedly reminded of their impotence against the virus, the invisible object of their fear. This reinforced their feeling of helplessness. Masks were the opposite of the will to power; they were a will to impotence.[19] Like security, risk is also an essential need of the soul: both must be kept in proportionate balance. Reckless risks should naturally be avoided. But the complete absence of risk produces in us a kind of boredom that paralyzes us almost as much as fear. Protecting ourselves from harm cannot mean the abolition of all risk.

As with the term *social* distancing instead of the more medical term *physical* distancing, I believe that a subtle language shift around masks signaled something significant. An interesting new term emerged during the pandemic: masks became *face coverings*. This is not a label doctors and nurses ever used to describe surgical masks, N95s, or other PPE. We do not call shirts *chest coverings* or socks *foot coverings* or shorts *genital coverings*. Why *face coverings*?

We were all compelled by various decrees and ubiquitous mechanisms of rigid enforcement to remain faceless in public, in some places for more than two years. *Merriam-Webster's Dictionary* defines "faceless" as "1a: lacking character or individuality: nondescript. // the *faceless* masses. 1b: not identified: anonymous. // a *faceless* accuser."[20] The dictionary on Apple devices similarly defines "faceless" as "remote and impersonal; anonymous: *the faceless bureaucrats who made the rules.*" Note the uncanny examples of usage provided by these dictionaries.

Might high-risk patients want to wear an N95 in settings of high transmission like hospitals? Might some masks have limited utility in some future pandemic in high-risk settings? Perhaps, though we should demand strong evidence of efficacy before mandating them anywhere. And we should realize that the widespread use of masks in public spaces inflicts harms that are no less serious for being difficult to precisely measure. They impair personal connections, alienating us from one another. Ask yourself: What must it have been like for a child to go through an entire day at school and not see a single person smile? Prolonged use of masks inflicts spiritual harms: they wound our souls.

If you are struggling with fear, and you have not done so already, consider uncovering your face. Refuse to remain *faceless* any longer. If this gives you some trepidation, it may be time to (literally) face your fear. I suggest we never again force one another to become nondescript entities, lacking character or individuality, unidentifiable, anonymous, remote, impersonal, or unseen. The face is not only the locus of human communication; it is the place where the personal dimension is most fully manifest. I recall moments during the pandemic when I experienced what I can only describe as "face hunger"—a strong desire to see the others around me in public spaces. Even when we were permitted to be together, we were forced to be *alone* together.

Until we are no longer faceless, we will remain impotent, alienated, incapable of making the necessary political or institutional changes. To borrow from the title of a modern retelling of the ancient myth of Cupid and Psyche: How can we become a flourishing society, how can we reestablish social bonds, how can we meet one another face to face, *till we have faces?*[21]

State of Normality

A 2019 video circulated online shows Hong Kong protestors approaching a thirty-foot-high facial recognition camera tower. With opened umbrellas to shield their faces from the camera, they sawed through the pole, pulled down the tower with ropes, stomped on the camera, and poured caustic liquid on the electronic components.[22] While this video cheered my heart, it clearly will take more than occasional outbursts of guerilla tactics to protect our privacy from the biosecurity surveillance regime.

Actions like this do suggest, however, that the paradigm of governance via the state of emergency—a frequent midwife to tyranny—is inherently unstable. Americans' widespread mistrust of elites, our skepticism toward tired bromides from prestige press, cloying celebrities, and scolding academicians, are salutary signs. For many people now see that those elites failed us: we know that the emperor stands naked before us, and he appears rather more foolish by the day.

Americans increasingly doubt the legitimacy of a regime that jumps from one proclaimed emergency to the next. As Stanford professor Russell Berman put it, "Let us not overstate the power of the emergency-declaring Leviathan that stands on feet of clay." He also wisely cautions, "Nor should we succumb to counterproductive extremism, which is used by the ideologues of the establishment to justify their emergency powers." Instead, he advises, "Let us be confident that their time is passing."[23] We can restore our privacy and our freedoms, though this will not happen automatically.

Similarly, although the problem of censorship by government, social media companies, and large media conglomerates is a difficult legal challenge, it is not insoluble. In April 2022 I tweeted, "Hey @elonmusk, can you also buy the WHO? It is currently owned by Bill Gates."[24] Elon replied with a wink and a pun: "I love Pinball Wizard!" with a link to that hit song by the band The Who.[25] Joking aside, we cannot rely merely on the goodwill of one billionaire to establish free speech on Twitter and other influential social media platforms. The problem requires legal solutions.

We can begin by insisting that our government respect our First Amendment right to free speech even when private corporations do not. In June of 2022, I submitted a declaration as an expert witness and a month later joined as a plaintiff in the case of *Schmitt & Landry v. Biden*.[26] Missouri attorney general Eric Schmitt and Louisiana attorney general Jeff Landry filed this lawsuit against President Biden and other top-ranking government officials for allegedly colluding with social media giants such as Facebook, Twitter, and YouTube to censor and suppress free speech. Our legal petition explains how the federal government has colluded with its social media companies to shadow-ban, deplatform, demonetize, de-boost, restrict content access, and suspend many speakers, both temporarily and permanently.

In other words the feds have been attempting to outsource their unconstitutional pandemic policy censorship to social media companies. Attorney General Schmitt commented, "We may have forced the Biden Administration to forego its Disinformation Governance Board, but there is still a very real threat to . . . Americans' right to free speech. The federal government must be halted from silencing any more Americans."[27] My expert-witness declaration described my personal experience of censorship on Twitter and LinkedIn, which we allege happened in direct response to Biden administration directives. Let's remember that the Constitution becomes a dead letter unless citizens continue to defend their constitutionally protected rights in the courts.

The economic predations of Davos Man will likewise prove challenging to reign in, given modernity's worship of the god Mammon and the staggering capital of gigantic finance firms like BlackRock ($10 trillion in assets under management) and private equity firms like Blackstone ($880 billion in assets). But we must find a way. I do not see any way we can simultaneously adopt digital IDs and central bank digital currencies while still protecting privacy and freedom. The only solution here is wholesale rejection of these centralized instruments—for these are designed precisely for surveillance and control. Whatever digital currencies we adopt need to be decentralized. Digital IDs are a Trojan horse that we should entirely reject.

The specifics of how to reestablish privacy, restore free speech, and reform global finance so that our economic systems operate on a human scale are problems that I confess lie outside my scope of expertise. My colleagues at the Ethics and Public Policy Center's "Big Tech Project" have promising proposals to address Big Tech censorship, and other thoughtful minds are working on privacy issues and economic reform. My hope is that this book at least convinces readers that serious and sustained efforts are needed in each of these domains, since they are all deeply implicated in the rise of the biomedical security state.

For my part I will limit my policy proposals here to reforms of scientific institutions and public health agencies, as well as legal reforms regarding declaring a state of emergency. These proposals are not meant to be comprehensive, and of course there are plenty of other policy ideas we should likewise consider. The important point is that we need a robust public conversation and broad agreement that there are indeed serious problems that call for robust reforms.

● ● ●

As a first political step toward a more human future, free people, acting together, must clearly demonstrate that there are strict limits to what citizens will accept under the rubric of a public health emergency. So far over the past three years, we have collectively delineated virtually no limits to these powers. It is past time for us to stand up together and pronounce a resounding "no" to the ongoing state of emergency.

As of this writing, in the summer of 2022, we are still living under a declared state of emergency at the federal level and in many states and counties, including my home state of California. That this state of exception has still not ended is an indictment of our political system's provisions for emergency powers. Americans who understand the implications should find this ongoing situation intolerable.

Covid is endemic: we cannot eradicate it, not ever. There are at least a dozen animal reservoirs—other species that get infected with this virus—so even if we eradicated it in humans (which is impossible), it would still circulate in other animals until it mutated sufficiently to reinfect our species. Yes, we have a population of vulnerable elderly that was never exposed to covid as children, so for now we need to help protect the elderly and continue to improve our early treatment regimens for those who get sick.

Every new covid season, like every new flu season, cannot be declared an emergency. We need to stop calling every new run of cases a "wave" and every new version a "variant of concern." We have new influenza strains every year, but we don't speak of an influenza "wave" with troubling new "variants" during flu season. SARS-CoV-2 will always be with us. But it is far from overwhelming our health care systems. There has not been a covid emergency for a long time now.

Must we have an available legal mechanism to declare states of emergency? Perhaps. Nature being what it is, we occasionally face disasters: floods, earthquakes, pestilence, and, yes, epidemics will come and go periodically. These will typically be localized and time-limited affairs. They may sometimes require the authorities, usually at the local or regional level, to declare a temporary state of emergency. But we cannot allow ongoing "emergencies" to define "the new normal." The state of exception needs to remain extremely exceptional.

This will require strict legal limits utilizing the same checks and balances the Constitution builds into our system of government. If we allow an executive or his appointee, whether the president, a governor, or a public health officer, to declare a state of emergency, the law needs to specify a strict time limit before this is subject to either legislative ratification or judicial review (or both). In an acute crisis, immediately after a devastating earthquake, for example, you don't want to wait for a vote. But the law can require a legislative vote sometime in the next week or two if the crisis continues. Several states already have such requirements. We can and should attempt, within reasonable levels of specificity, to define in law thresholds for what constitutes an emergency—thresholds that would allow for periodic judicial review.

The executive typically assumes additional powers in the state of emergency. Thus, the executive branch should not be the sole authority responsible for continuing this state of emergency beyond strict time limits. To start with, we should rescind the 2013 National Defense Act, the federal law that permitted the $1 billion federal expenditure on vaccine advertisements and permitted governors to dictate terms to legacy media and social media regarding "misinformation" content. Wiser legal minds than mine can hammer out the other details, but the basic principles of separation of powers and legislative or judicial checks and balances can minimize the possibility of an endless state of emergency. This principle, wisely applied, can also interrupt the toxic pattern of jumping from one emergent crisis to the next, which has increasingly characterized our political life since World War II and was turbocharged during the last three years.

In July 2022, for example, President Biden asked his staff to see if he "has the authority" to declare a public health emergency to address abortion access. This move would release additional funding and give federal health officials more power to respond to state-level abortion restrictions, following the Supreme Court's overturning of *Roe v. Wade*.[28] As a constitutional matter, the Supreme Court in *Dobbs* returned the issue of abortion to the states. Biden's bid to declare a state of emergency for abortion access attempts to unilaterally transfer authority on this issue from the states back to the federal government, specifically to his own executive branch. Leveraging the state-of-exception legal mechanism for this controversial issue would circumvent the Constitution's specified delegation of powers.

If we choose to maintain provisions for states of emergencies in our legal frameworks, we should demand at least some evidence that these in fact help during times of emergencies. There is surprisingly little research supporting this notion. One study of various emergency constitutions found, contrary to expectations, that "the more advantages emergency constitutions confer to the executive, the higher the number of people killed as a consequence of a natural disaster, controlling for its severity." Since this was an unanticipated result, the authors explored several possible explanations, and concluded: "The most plausible [explanation] being that governments use natural disasters as a pretext to enhance their power."[29] Gosh, who would have thought?

We should also maintain *permanent* limits on the state of exception. In a sane society, there are human and spiritual goods that should never be relinquished, even—one might say especially—under extraordinary circumstances. The people most responsible for reminding of us of this—with a few notable exceptions—failed during the pandemic. All too many religious leaders and clergy unfortunately showed themselves during the pandemic to be willing chaplains to the new technocracy. It is time for them to reassert their proper scope of spiritual authority over the communities entrusted to their care.

Institutional Reforms

Our public health agencies, scientific institutions, and medical systems also failed us, full stop. It will take decades to rebuild public trust in these institutions. Many people, including highly educated professionals, no longer want to see a physician; some don't want to go to a hospital ever again. People don't know where to turn anymore for credible information about medicine or public health. While we masked up, the pandemic itself was a kind of *unmasking*, in the sense that it revealed the degree to which many of our institutions had already decayed from within. These institutions will take a generation or more to rebuild. In many instances, it will be more productive to build entirely new institutions rather than try to repair the old rotted-out structures.

The necessary reforms of our HHS bureaucracies—the NIH, CDC, FDA—may not be feasible anytime soon, given the entrenched interests of the administrative state and the tendency for these agencies to become ends in themselves. New directors at the helm—even competent, honest, and well-intentioned leaders—may simply not be able to reign in the entrenched corrosive tendencies or disentangle the deeply rooted conflicts of interest.

A professor friend at one of the Ivy League medical schools once remarked to me that the university eats its own young. The Leviathan administrative state—what some have dubbed the deep state—likewise eats its own young. In the absence of wholesale reform, we at least need to rein in the monolithic power of our public health agencies.

Quite obviously, there needs to be a bipartisan congressional investigation of our entire pandemic response. I suggest also that we require the Senate ratify the president's appointment of three-letter agency directors, with strict limits on how long any single person can remain in that position. In the second chapter, I briefly discussed the regulatory capture of these agencies by pharmaceutical companies and related economic interests. We must erect robust firewalls to mitigate these obvious financial conflicts of interest. All NIH, CDC, and FDA regulators should be entirely free from pharma funding.

"Public-private partnerships" in this realm are a euphemism for corruption and agency capture, a thin veneer for corporatism. Agency funding must come directly from the government, with robust congressional oversight, period. Pharmaceutical companies need to be liable for safety problems with their vaccines just as they are for the medications they produce. Once their indemnity is revoked, these companies will produce safer products that they more adequately test for safety before marketing.

We also need to shut and lock the revolving door between industry and pharma. Regulators must have a long tail on their contract (fifteen years would not be too long) that prevents them from working for the companies they only recently regulated. Legal mechanisms, such as noncompete clauses used in other industries, can be helpful here. Obviously, pharmaceutical company executives should never move from industry into positions within regulatory agencies. My friend Robert Malone has cogently argued that the CDC and NIH foundations, whose boards are populated with pharmaceutical company executives, need to be decommissioned immediately. Private donations cannot be permitted to influence government decisions about research funding or public health policy. Malone points out that moneyed interests are intentionally using these foundations to bypass federal laws designed to limit undue corporate influence on federal decision-making.[30]

Pharmaceutical companies currently conduct their own clinical trials on their products, which creates potential problems. The clinical trials necessary for FDA authorization need to be funded publicly and conducted by researchers who are free of financial ties to pharmaceutical companies. Funding could come from taxing pharma companies on profits. All the de-identified data from clinical trials, and not just the final published papers, should be made publicly available for independent analysis in a database maintained by the FDA. This was the purpose of our FOIA request for the Pfizer vaccine data, as described in the second chapter, but it should not require expensive private legal action from concerned citizens to access this kind of data.

The CDC should immediately be split into two separate entities housing its two distinct functions. On the one hand, the CDC is now responsible for collecting, synthesizing, and publishing epidemiological data from the individual states—a scientific data-gathering function. This data is crucial for medical and public health researchers around the country. On the other hand, the CDC is also responsible for making public health recommendations and policies—an inescapably political function. At times, these two functions are in tension or clear conflict. For example the CDC stopped or slowed the publication of data on the pandemic in 2021 and 2022 (its scientific function), citing worries that the data might increase "vaccine hesitancy" (its policy function).

These distinct functions should be separated into two entirely separate agencies that operate with a firewall between them. We need a national epidemiological agency responsible only for publishing data and required by law to publish all the data gathered from states and other sources. Then we can have a separate agency responsible for public health and policy recommendations. Housing these functions under the same roof created a tangle of unnecessary problems during the pandemic.

Regarding the publication and dissemination of scientific research, there is also need for major reforms. Many specialized areas of scientific research involve a small community of researchers, where the same senior academics peer-review papers for publication, serve as editors at the most prestigious journals, review NIH grant requests, vote on promotion for academic colleagues, and write letters of recommendation for colleagues seeking tenure at other institutions. The concept of peer review sounds sensible enough, but there are serious downsides to the current system. As it is now configured, the same small group of senior researchers often acts as gatekeepers for all the avenues necessary for academic advancement in science: publication, research funding, promotion, and tenure.

This creates a culture in which junior faculty are often reluctant to challenge the consensus of the senior gatekeepers out of concern for harming their academic careers. We'd like to believe that all scientists are open-minded and welcome intellectual debate and challenge. In practice there are strong centralizing trends within scientific institutions that encourage groupthink. Orthodoxies are often driven by entrenched interests or by strong personalities who do not like their prestige or influence challenged by young upstarts or dissidents within the ranks. Alas, we cannot escape human nature, with all its frailty and folly, and scientific research is nothing if not a human enterprise.

The currently cumbersome and often biased process of anonymous peer review should be replaced with an open peer-review system. Open peer-review reports, with the review author's name listed, could be published alongside the relevant paper. These ancillary commentaries can critique the methodology, contextualize the research, or explain the salience and limitations of the original paper's findings. Or they can present reasons why the published paper is plain wrong and without merit. Critical readers can read both and draw their own conclusions. Those who advance sound and accurate research findings will not fear open discussion, critique, and debate. Those who feel challenged by new research findings will have to state publicly why their interlocutors got it wrong.

To address data mining and statistical spinning of results, there are already proposals within the scientific community to require the posting of study methodology prior to a study's being conducted. This prevents post hoc changes to trial endpoints and discourages statistical games to fish for findings that can compromise the integrity of study design and published trial results. It is a scandal that the findings in roughly 85 percent of published biomedical research cannot be subsequently reproduced by other researchers.[31] The replication crisis in medical research—which is now well known—should result in major reforms to improve the rigor, quality, and reproducibility of published scientific findings. I am a friend, not an enemy, of science. I say this not as the little boy pointing to the naked emperor, but as someone at a party discreetly whispering to a friend that he would do well to zip up his fly.

Academia has a role here: the "publish or perish" mandate for faculty results in the publication of mountains of half-baked "research" that is little better than rubbish, and the consequent proliferation of "peer-reviewed" journals that publish sloppy or irrelevant research that nobody reads or cites. Academic advancement needs to rest upon quality, not quantity, and weigh other contributions of faculty (teaching, clinical work, university service, community outreach) beyond publishing papers. Like our public health agencies, scientific journals must stop taking payments from pharma, including advertising and the sale of reprints. This may require additional public funding to support peer-reviewed journals, but there are other potential solutions that we will see in a moment that won't strain the public purse.

My colleague Martin Kulldorff, a former Harvard epidemiologist now at the Brownstone Institute, was among the most sane and sensible scientific voices during the pandemic. He pointed out that during covid some of the best pandemic research did not come from the United States, the United Kingdom, or other places considered "the powerhouses" of science. It came instead from places like Qatar, Israel, Denmark, Sweden, and Iceland. Kulldorff argues that one reason is that scientists in these countries are somewhat removed from the dominant "cartels" that control scientific institutions in the powerhouse nations: these countries' scientific institutions are more on the periphery, especially when it comes to seeking funding for research.

This led, paradoxically, not to marginal research but innovative and important contributions that advanced our understanding of the pandemic. These places often did the research that we should have done but were not doing. The most significant studies on covid treatments, on natural immunity, and on vaccine efficacy came mostly from outside the United States and the United Kingdom. Anyone who has studied the history of science and medicine will realize that this is not unusual: innovation and major advances typically come from the creative periphery, not from the sclerotic and entrenched center.

To prevent a small cabal of editors at the major medical journals from controlling what gets published, Kulldorff has proposed that each university should have its own journal, which would publish the work of its own research faculty. Broad participation, with the wider scientific community (not just invited reviewers) able to submit open peer-review commentaries, would help prevent some of the editorial cherry-picking that limits the scientific voices. In this revised system, papers rise in significance based not on which journal they are published in—the most "prestigious" science journals published plenty of nonsense during the pandemic, after all—but on the number of citations they receive and the influence the papers have on advancing subsequent work and contributing to the field over time. As with books that stay in print for decades or centuries and thereby become classics, good papers will be remembered, and shoddy ones will eventually be forgotten.

Funding for scientific research likewise cannot be controlled by a small group of insiders at the NIH, many of whom stay in power for decades, acting like presidents in a banana republic who never face serious reelection challenges. The current system of NIH sinecure allows the likes of Anthony Fauci to wield enormous power over primary investigators and their teams of university researchers, permitting one man to shape the entire research agenda of infectious disease for a generation or more. There are many potential approaches to breaking up this monopoly.

For my part I suggest federal block grants to states to fund scientific research, so that each state has its own version of an NIH. Instead of one NIH we could have fifty SIHs—State Institutes of Health. Each state could compete for researchers by offering attractive grants, or perhaps could carve out specific niches within the enormous enterprise of scientific research, focusing on problems or diseases that impact its citizens. Alaska could fund research on hypothermia, Hawaii on sunstroke, Washington on seasonal affective disorder, and so on. Nothing in this system would prevent several states from partnering to co-fund large research projects that require greater resources or impact larger regions.

Doctors need to be free again, as we had always been until the pandemic, to prescribe off-label or repurposed drugs at our discretion. This has long been permitted under federal law and is a routine practice in every branch of medicine. Pharmacies or hospitals should never be permitted to refuse to fill prescriptions from licensed physicians who have done an appropriate medical evaluation. My friend and colleague Dr. Pierre Kory has a lot more to say on this score, and I recommend we pay attention. Physicians need discretionary latitude to individualize care for specific patients. Every patient, like every person, is unique and unrepeatable. Innovations and data from real-time experiences of frontline doctors in the trenches are every bit as necessary when treating a new pathogen as ivory tower research. The two realms need to reinforce and influence each other. We need to let doctors once again be doctors.

Informed consent must be restored to a central place in medical ethics. But we can only have informed consent if we have accurate information presented to the public. This is among the reasons that a free and independent media is so vital. I hope it is obvious why we need a free press, including a free scientific press, not subject to coercion from government or private interests. Without this, it's game over.

Censorship and science are utterly incompatible. The rampant conflicts of interest in media are a difficult problem to solve, given the role of advertising and the media's financial temptation to publish clickbait.

One crucial step, however, is to stop allowing direct-to-consumer advertising of pharmaceutical products. Media conglomerates will need to go elsewhere to find giant pots of advertising dollars, and pharma can redirect that marketing money to research and development. As already mentioned, we are only one of two countries in the world that permits "ask your doctor about . . ." ads on television and radio. When they see these for the first time, people in other countries rightly think these commercials are crazy. Doctors are the gatekeepers for prescription drugs: that's why we go through at least seven postgraduate years of training before board certification. There are reasons prescription drugs are not available over the counter or by mail order. Advertising medications on television is not just gauche and in poor taste; it's harmful to medicine and detrimental to the public good.

Many other proposals have been floated by thoughtful critics of the current crisis in science and medicine. The replication crisis—the demonstrated inability of most scientific findings to be replicated in subsequent studies—has already spurred thinking in this area. Hubris and outsized egos undermine rigorous science, though these remain perennial temptations. Scientists are human, alas, all too human. But there are thoughtful ways to place checks in the system, to minimize perverse incentives and to dampen the untoward effects of human greed, pride, vanity, and envy in science.

We can argue endlessly about the pros and cons of specific proposals, and we should. But we need to start with a basic agreement that something is broken, indeed very badly broken, in our scientific, medical, and public health institutions. We have serious problems requiring deep reforms to address. We can and should debate the best prescriptions to address this disease, but I hope we can at least find broad agreement on the diagnosis.

The Cunning of Reason

Václav Havel, a playwright, essayist, and political dissident, was elected president of the Czech Republic following the fall of the Soviet empire. Unlike most politicians—Lincoln and Churchill being other notable exceptions—Havel wrote beautiful prose. In a brilliant essay, "Politics and Conscience," Havel reflected on the modern political situation in light of the changes he had lived through in Eastern Europe. He noted that rulers and leaders were once personalities in their own right, "with particular human faces, still in some sense personally responsible for their deeds, good and ill," regardless of how they came to occupy positions of power.

In modern times, however, real political personalities have been replaced by the manager, the bureaucrat, the apparatchik, the technocrat: "a professional ruler, manipulator, and expert in the techniques of management, manipulation, and obfuscation, filling a depersonalized intersection of functional relations." These rulers are themselves a "cog in the machinery of state caught up in a predetermined role." Today's professional ruler is the unaware instrument of anonymous powers, "legitimized by science, cybernetics, ideology, law, abstraction, and objectivity—that is, by everything except personal responsibility to human beings as persons and neighbors."[32] Remove the technocrat's public mask and underneath you see . . . nothing. This is the faceless instrument managing the biomedical security state.

As Havel wrote, "Behind his judicious mask and affected diction there is not a trace of a human being rooted in the order of the natural world by his loves, passions, interests, personal opinions, hatred, courage, or cruelty." All this he locks away in his private room. "If we glimpse anything at all behind the mask, it will be only the more or less competent technician of power." The result, Havel explains, is that "states grow ever more machinelike; people are transformed into statistical choruses of voters, producers, consumers, patients, tourists, or soldiers."[33] In our time, both rulers and ruled are subsumed into this machine made of human parts.

Other contemporary thinkers, from Alasdair MacIntyre to Philip Rieff, have likewise described this amoral manager, this calculating therapeutic technocrat, as the archetypal ruler of our time. In MacIntyre's description the manager treats ends as given, as outside his scope of competence, always beyond the range of his responsibilities. His exclusive concern is with technique, with efficient means toward predetermined ends. Rationality is only purely instrumental. The cunning of reason serves either private interest, self-seeking designs, or external interests determined by powers outside his purview. The technocrat just follows orders.

The goals come prepackaged and ready-made, and the politician as manager can relinquish responsibility for pursuing those ends. Virtually all our leaders abdicated responsibility during the pandemic in favor of what "The Experts" told them, though it must be admitted these were handpicked experts who advocated policies to their liking. Anyone not on board was vilified as "anti-science" or a "pandemic denier." We saw this character type directing our entire pandemic response from the beginning. The pure bureaucrat literally *becomes* the bureaucracy, exercising, as I have said, enormous power with no locus of responsibility.

Any cure for this will require that we first hold our leaders accountable for their decisions. Hiding behind "The Science" or "The Experts," thereby abdicating responsibility, cannot continue as the preferred mode of our political life. Decisions during a pandemic are never read off directly from a few charts and graphs. Yes, rulers should be informed by input from various domains of expertise. Countless charts and graphs, showing not just the epidemiology of covid but presenting input from a hundred other disciplines, are potentially relevant.

Even with all this, however, a thousand more imponderables come into play when considering a specific policy decision like lockdowns or mass vaccination—or the decision about whether a declared state of emergency is justified in the first place. Making consequential judgments in the face of uncertainty is admittedly difficult. We can forgive mistakes made in real time, but on condition that mistakes are acknowledged and course corrections made. We should not, however, continue to tolerate political decision-makers who wash their hands of responsibility for their decisions.

Specific individuals—not some fictitious monolithic "Science"—made the public policy decisions that I critiqued in this book. Most of our consequential pandemic decisions were disastrous, so disastrous it's difficult to wrap one's head around the carnage they caused. Our leaders are responsible. Indeed, we are all, to one degree or another, responsible—every single one of us—as citizens of this supposedly representative democracy. I allowed this to happen, you allowed it, and they allowed it. This is on us. In a democratic republic we get the rulers we deserve.

• • •

As we near the end of this book, the reader who has persevered this far will permit me one last brief philosophical detour. As we discussed at the close of the previous chapter, beginning with Plato, the predominant strand of philosophy in the West has affirmed that man participates in a universal form of rationality—a transcendent *logos* (a rich Greek concept simultaneously signifying reason, word, order, and intelligibility) that informs all of reality. Our shared participation in a universal reason is the precondition for pursuing scientific truths, communicating them, and understanding them.

Given this shared participation, we can deliberate and debate one another in a common pursuit of truth. If we are humble and persevering, we can correct our mistakes, and we can attempt—however imperfectly—to place the truth above our own narrow or selfish interests. Reason can become more than mere cunning, more than an instrumental tool of power. You and I may not agree, but I maintain respect and regard for you as a person—as someone capable of seeking, discovering, and, hopefully, embracing the truth once it is known. Each of us participates in the *logos* only imperfectly, and thus the pursuit of truth is a never-ending and ongoing project. None of us individually or as a clique have a monopoly on reason.

A strand of modern rationalist philosophy tracing back five hundred years and culminating in Marx as its unsurpassed representative presents us with a very different view of human rationality. Following Hegel, Marx affirmed that history inevitably moves towards the liberation of mankind. But this axiom entailed that Marx abandon the search for truth in favor of the search for what is practically effective, for what will move history toward its fulfillment. As Marx famously put it, other philosophers have merely understood the world, but the point is to change it. It was not as though Marx just got restless and wanted to get out of the armchair where he was theorizing to put his philosophical ideas into practice. Underlying his remark is a radically redefined concept of truth and knowledge.

In his conception man is no longer measured by reason—by truth, reality, the cosmos, God, or anything else that might transcend us. Instead, man is the measure of reason—and reason is merely an instrumentally useful tool for achieving purely human aims. For Marx, rationality does not discover the truth of things. Rationality is instead the engine of activity that transforms the material world—reason is an agent of "praxis," to use the Marxist term. Human reason does not *comprehend* truth by grasping the world as it is; indeed, truth is not something "out there" that we *discover*. On this view, reason instead *creates* truth by changing the world through revolutionary action. Truth is literally *what we make.*

Recall Marx's first principle: that history moves in a deterministic direction, fueled by purely material factors and social conditions. "Ideas" are just the foam on the wave of history—a kind of "superstructure" stemming entirely from the material-social-economic forces operating underneath. There is thus no change of man's ideas without a change in these material-social forces. For Marx, history is not driven by ideas, which have no causal power, but purely by impersonal material and economic forces. How this notion squares with the idea that history is moving toward fulfillment in a future utopia is a serious problem for Marx, but set that aside for the moment.

One corollary of this—and this brings us into direct contact with the transhumanist project—is that Marx was the first philosopher to deny that there is such a thing as human nature. There is no *given* for man: humanity is simply what we *make* ourselves. Freedom in this view requires not just *self-determination* but radical *self-creation*. The odyssey of history must lead to a divinized self-creating man who is pure greatness, the master of his own destiny. Man is divinized not by grace or anything from above; he is divinized by his own activity, his own human effort to remake the political and material order.

Now, we quite obviously cannot each create ourselves individually—after all, every individual was born from a mother and has a father and is dependent. Each of us has a belly button. But because we are purely the product of material and economic forces, Marx affirms the idea of *social* self-creation: we create ourselves anew through our economic and political activity, by means of which we reconstruct the world entirely from scratch. By radically remaking the material world, we radically remake our humanity. Thus, a total revolution, with a complete rupture from all previous history, is capable of totally refashioning mankind—a new creation *ex nihilo*.

Now, here is the practical upshot of this philosophy. According to this view, science and technology are the tools that make our self-creation possible. Marx would not say that his was a philosophy that comprehends the world, but a philosophy that becomes the world. Rationality is instrumentally useful to manipulate reality, to remake things in my own image. This is the cunning of reason: ideas are merely productive tools, not reflections of some transcendent truth. Indeed, for Marx, any idea that is true for everyone could only be enslaving. Hence the radical relativism characteristic of his many descendants, among whom are the transhumanists.

By contrast, according to the classical Platonic idea of rationality, human beings can reason and deliberate together in a shared pursuit.

Reason is not just instrumental; it is contemplative. Knowledge is intrinsically good for its own sake. This conception of the "light of reason" is represented in the motto of the University of California, emblazoned over an open book on the university's logo: *Fiat Lux*—let there be light. The light of the human intellect can come to know the world. Indeed, creation itself is knowable precisely because it also participates in the *logos*. Reality has an ordered, intelligible structure, comprehensible to the human mind and capable of being described by, for example, the laws of physics and other scientific disciplines. The light of reason gently compels assent without violating our freedom. When we "see" that $2 + 2 = 4$, we freely assent to this proposition without the slightest hint of coercion.

And here we come to the point. Many of us during the pandemic puzzled over why data and evidence did not seem to put a dent in some people's convictions about covid or our public policies. Perhaps this was because we had implicit Platonists (understanding that term broadly) trying to communicate with implicit Marxists (also understood broadly, regardless of whether they had read a word of Marx). Those who had a shared-participatory view of reason were talking past those who had an instrumental-material view of rationality. The light of reason could find no purchase with the cunning of reason. The twain could not possibly meet. The very same words carried two entirely different meanings. Is truth something we discover in the world, or is truth what we ourselves create entirely by our will to power? People who disagree on this foundational question cannot engage in a fruitful debate about science or evidence.

These two fundamental streams, which run through ancient and modern philosophy, present us with a basic choice between *persuasion* and *force*. Writing in the wake of the devastation of World War II and just before her death, Simone Weil put the matter this way in a magnificent book called *The Need for Roots*: "Either we must perceive at work in the universe, alongside force, a principle of a different kind, or else we must recognize force as being the unique and sovereign ruler over human relations also." Reflecting on the Marxist and Fascist ideologies that had just torn the world apart, she wrote, "The great instigators of violence have encouraged themselves with the thought of how blind, mechanical force is sovereign throughout the whole universe."[34]

As you might suspect, dear reader, I am an unabashed Platonist—at least in the broad sense of the term sketched here. The light of reasoned persuasion, which gently compels assent without compromising our freedom, is our only way forward. Force—and its close cousins, censorship and slander—have no place in public discourse.

I encourage you to learn everything you can from people with expertise in relevant scientific disciplines. Consider their advice and their input. But remember also that each one of us is in possession of logic, common sense, and the capacity for shared rationality. Therefore, do not outsource your logic, common sense, and rationality to "experts." Every person of sound mind shares this human capacity for contact with reality. You too can perceive the truth and choose to adhere to it unconditionally. You too can discern and reject falsehood and error. Truth is not the exclusive province of a Gnostic, technocratic elite.

Each of us must do the hard work to pursue the truth and to grasp it, making it our own. Groupthink is a contradiction, for groups do not have thoughts. Again, we can cite Weil on the topic of freedom of opinion and its consequences for ethical action: "The intelligence is defeated as soon as the expression of one's thoughts is preceded, explicitly or implicitly, by the little word 'we.' And when the light of the intelligence grows dim, it is not very long before the love of good becomes lost."[35]

You may not be an expert in virology or epidemiology or any other scientific discipline. But this is of little consequence: you can spot a blatant contradiction, you can see when things don't add up, you can reason logically from premises to conclusions. You are perfectly capable of recognizing that even science is subject to extrinsic fashions, and that "consensus" judgments are oftentimes swayed by all-too-human motivations. I passionately love science. I have loved studying it and practicing it from my earliest years. Science is a wondrous enterprise, a very noble and good pursuit.

But science will fail us the moment we turn it into an idol. And scientists will fail us the moment we turn them into oracles.

The Need for Roots

Augusto Del Noce, the prescient Italian philosopher we met at the end of the opening chapter, argued that our scientistic-technocratic society "cannot be surpassed through a revolution, but only by restoring the religious dimension and the moral authority of values."[36] To be clear, he drew a distinction between what he called the religious dimension and religion: the *religious dimension is the questions* to which revealed religion proposes answers. These questions include, among others, Why am I here? What is the purpose of my life? What is my final destiny? What constitutes a flourishing society? Why is there something rather than nothing? Where are we now and how did we get here?

The scientistic-technocratic society will not be surpassed without restoring these questions and respecting the moral authority of enduring ethical values. In our affluent society focused on purely material well-being, where reason is reduced to an instrumental role, we must regain the capacity to ask these questions and wrestle with the answers. If the central feature of all totalitarianisms is the inability to pose questions like these—the forced exclusion of certain questions from the realm of rational discourse—we can grasp the importance of keeping these questions always publicly alive, not merely tucked away in some remote corner of our private lives.

To meet the challenges we face, we need not seek to become new men. We need not seek new gods, certainly not new divinities of our own creation, which are bound to turn on us in the end. Here in the aftermath of the past three years, among the ruins that both the virus and our response to it have wrought, we need to build a more rooted human future. Our problems are not superficial, and they did not develop overnight. We need to be thinking now in hundred-year increments. This entails a willingness to plant seeds that we may not see germinate in our lifetime.

Many people have asked me, since I clearly don't like the pandemic politics in California, why don't I move to another state that took a different approach to covid? I often answer that what happens in California tends to spread to other states—we are the tip of the spear, so to speak—and so I want to stay and fight for sanity here. This is true, but the more important part of my answer is simpler. I stay here because this is my home. I grew up in the Pacific Northwest, went to college in the Midwest, and attended medical school on the East Coast. But I have now lived in California longer than anywhere else. My family and I have put down roots here.

We all have a deep human need for rootedness. In today's world, characterized by cosmopolitan mobility, instantaneous digital communication, and global travel, this need is often harder to recognize. I am convinced, however, that without being rooted we have no chance of resisting the rising biomedical security state. A tree can withstand strong winds only if it has put down strong roots. This does not mean, of course, that one necessarily stays put where one happens to reside. In Weil's description, "A human being has roots by virtue of his real, active and natural participation in the life of a community which preserves in living shape certain particular treasures of the past and certain particular expectations for the future."[37]

It is precisely this participation in the life of a community that we were denied during covid. Whether or not we got sick with the virus, all of us are now afflicted to some extent with the disease of uprootedness. The misfortune of unemployment, which exploded due to pandemic policies that regarded scores of workers as expendable, is certainly among the more severe forms of uprootedness—for dignified work is a basic human need. "The contemporary form of true greatness," Weil wrote, "lies in a civilization founded upon the spirituality of work."[38] Contrary to some contemporary gurus, the profound uprootedness characteristic of unemployment cannot be cured or even palliated by video games, online porn, or recreational drugs. Not only is this an inhumane proposal, but the uprootedness of one class will inevitably spread like a cancer to other sectors of society.

The maniacal desire for pecuniary gain, which drove much of our pandemic response, also destroys human roots. A steady diet of mass media propaganda, driven by financial interests or political expedients instead of a dispassionate search for truth, constitutes another acid that erodes our roots. We have thrown our past away, "just like a child picking off the petals of a rose,"[39] trading it for a series of "instants" flickering across our screens. This loss of our past, the erasure of our sense of history, also contributes to our uprootedness. This is among the reasons I began this book with a bit of history in the prologue.

The sad fact that so many of us fell for cheap propaganda during the pandemic suggests that our contemporary systems of education likewise contribute to our lack of roots. Commenting on the topic of propaganda, Hitler said that brute force is unable to prevail over ideas if it is alone, but it easily manages to prevail by taking into itself a few ideas, no matter how base or simplistic. Truly educated people—and I am referring to a full human education of the emotions and passions, of the conscience as well as the intellect—do not fall for these cheap parlor tricks. This is far from the kind of education we offer the young, and so the problem runs very deep in our culture. The solution to this problem must begin in kindergarten. Indeed, it begins in the home even before kindergarten.

Uprootedness tends to be a self-propagating disease. As Weil observed, for people who are uprooted there remain only two possible behavioral responses: "Either to fall into a spiritual lethargy resembling death, like the majority of the slaves in the days of the Roman Empire, or to hurl themselves into some form of activity necessarily designed to uproot, often by the most violent methods, those who are not yet uprooted, or only partly so."[40] Unless we reestablish roots in real human communities, we are liable to fall prey to one or another of these destructive tendencies—spiritual lethargy or corrosive activism. It is no accident that terrorists and drug dealers recruit among the uprooted. Perhaps some corporate C-suites and academic institutions do as well.

If I am correct—that the need for roots is necessary for human flourishing in a more human future—this means *every one of us has a part to play in creating that future.* None of us is helpless to do something, for each of us can reach out to our friends and neighbors and begin to build real forms of rooted communities, however simple and humble these first gatherings or initiatives might be. If you begin to connect to others face to face, to rebuild friendships, to repair family relationships, to contribute to your neighborhood, your community, or to a worthy cause with your personal labor and your devotion, you are helping to build this future. You need be neither an expert nor a person with elevated power and position. You can simply start small—small is beautiful. As suggested in the previous section, we need to regain a sense of personal agency if we want to build a richly textured human future, and we need to demand personal agency and responsibility from our leaders.

In January 2021 I sat down for an interview with the producer of the *Planet Lockdown* documentary series. Toward the end of the interview, he asked me two questions that seem fitting for the conclusion of this book. After I sketched for him the outlines of the biomedical security state, I cautioned that this world is coming soon if we don't wake up from our sleepwalking and start to push back. He then asked me, "What do you think people have to lose by resisting these things?" I gave the following answer:

> People have a lot to lose by resisting. I lost my job. You may be called names. You might be vilified by certain people. You may lose friendships and relationships if you stand up, put a stake in the ground, and behave differently—if you don't continue to "go along to get along." But you have everything to gain. There's nothing better than waking up with a clear conscience every day. There's nothing better than living your life in such a way that you can tell your

children or your grandchildren, your nieces or nephews—the next generation—that when this thing was being rolled out, I tried to stand up against it. I was one of the few that took a stand—who recognized what was percolating, what was developing, saw what was coming, and said, "No, I'm not going to be a part of that."

I think that's what we need right now. We need people to look within themselves, to examine their conscience and decide where they're going to put that stake in the ground, where they will draw the line in the sand, and then we need people of moral courage to stand strong even in the face of countervailing winds and pressures. So, you have something to lose if you do that, but you have everything to gain.

Many people from all over the world reached out to encourage me after I took a stand against the university's vaccine mandate. Often, they would tell me that I was on the "right side of history." I appreciated the sentiment and encouragement, understanding them to mean that some-day people would recognize that I did the right thing and that my cause was just. But strictly speaking, history does not have sides. There is no invisible hand operating within history that guarantees that what is best in any given period will be transmitted to posterity or that truth will eventually prevail. Sometimes truths are buried, and they remain forever buried, never coming to light. Sometimes injustices are never rectified in this world.

Contrary to Hegel and, I'm sorry to say it, Martin Luther King Jr., the arc of history does not inevitably bend toward justice. Just as force is not a machine that automatically produces justice, so also the unfolding of history does not automatically produce justice. The ethics of the "direction of history" is false precisely because history does not have a predetermined direction. The myth of inevitable moral progress is just that—a myth, evident from the rise and fall of civilizations and empires and the emergence of new evils that must be met and minimized in every generation. The future will not inevitably be better than the present or the past. And wherever pure force rules as sovereign, justice is an unreal chimera, always out of reach.

So, I don't believe in a progressive direction of history. I don't believe that any coming revolution—whether technological or political—will bring about a future utopia. But the opposite of this kind of historical determinism is not nihilism; it is the idea of Providence. This idea posits that we are characters in a larger ongoing drama that unfolds in history. We are actors on the stage, characters in a story scripted by another writer-director; we are musicians in a symphony orchestrated by another conductor. I am fond of the seventeenth-century philosopher Giambattista Vico's classic definition of Providence:

> It is true that men have themselves made this world of nations ... but this world without doubt has issued from a mind often diverse, at times quite contrary, and always superior to the particular ends that men had proposed to themselves; which narrow ends, made to serve wider ends, it has always employed to preserve the human race upon this earth.[41]

We cannot foresee all ends and we cannot predict all outcomes. Even the wisest see only dimly into the near future. It is thus a profound consolation to believe that our narrow purposes in our tiny moment of history serve wider purposes that we cannot fully comprehend. All we can do is play our modest part as actors in the wider historical drama. There is no guarantee that we will succeed individually or collectively; but if we refuse to play our part, we are sure to fail. Success is always provisional, but success is not finally our responsibility anyways. As T. S. Eliot put it in his *Four Quartets*, which I cited in the opening chapter: "For us there is only the trying. The rest is not our business."

That force cannot produce justice does not mean that justice is unreal: it is real enough in the hearts of people of goodwill. It's an ideal that, however much some might try, cannot be eradicated. Weil argued,

"If justice is inerasable from the heart of Man," even if science alone cannot discover it, "it must have a reality in this world. It is science, then, which is mistaken."[42] Or more precisely, it is the ideology that scientific knowledge is the only form of true knowledge—scientism—that is mistaken. The realm of moral knowledge is no less real, and it can never be completely forgotten or erased.

In closing, I would like to return to the documentary interview I cited above. After asking me what people stand to lose by resisting the biomedical security state, the interviewer closed with this question: "What final words do you have to help others through this?" I will conclude this book with the same response I gave that day—an answer that came to me in that moment without any forethought:

> History is not set in stone. The future is not predetermined by the past. History is made by the decisions of individuals. There are social, there are economic, there are political, there are all kinds of other forces at work that no doubt shape human history and shape our collective actions. But ultimately, human beings are free and rational individuals who can discern the good, who can freely choose the good, or who can choose to pursue other paths. So, my advice is to remember that the future is not set in stone. The future really depends on what we do now. And I think all of us want to wake up in ten, twenty, thirty years and be able to tell the next generation that we stood up and did everything in our power—regardless of the outcome—to make sure that we were handing on a world to them that was humane, that was livable, that was just, and that was free.[43]

Now it's time for us to go to work.

Seattle, 2030

*We must always tell what we see. Above all, and this is
more difficult, we must always see what we see.*

—*Charles Péguy*

The year is 2030 and you are living with your wife and children in
Seattle, Washington.[1]

The world has changed since the covid pandemic. Globally, tensions
have escalated between the United States and China. There's constant
chatter among conservative talking heads that we are engaged in a new
cold war. A few even worry about escalation to a hot war as China's
military capabilities continue to expand, but you are not convinced.
China is not Russia, after all—China may be authoritarian, but it is not
some rogue state led by a crazy demagogue. Following Russia's failed
invasion of Ukraine, aside from sporadic outbreaks of ethnic conflict in
India and Africa, the world has not seen another major international
conflict since the covid pandemic ended.

While a few commentators maintain, and many political satirists
joke, that politicians should be subject to automation like so many other
industries—"Bots Can Govern Us Better!" the meme proclaims—the
level of citizens' trust in government has generally improved since the
days of covid. Most align with the centrist position that embraces scientific management via AI-enhanced governance without doing away

entirely with elected officials. This position was articulated a dozen years ago in a 2018 paper from the World Economic Forum:

> For the time being, it seems neither possible nor optimal for robots to replace government leaders, despite the clear imperfections displayed by the latter group. . . . Ultimately, a more realistic and desirable scenario is one in which AI and automation are neither competitors nor substitutes to humans, but tools that government leaders can engage effectively and sometimes defer to, in order to make better, fairer and more inclusive decisions.[2]

Across the border in Canada, French-speaking Québécois radicals are agitating again, arguing that since the Québécois nation was recognized by the Canadian House of Commons in 2006, they have a right to territorial sovereignty. Prime Minister Justin Trudeau, who was re-elected after spending a term out of office, maintains that the 2006 parliamentary resolution employed a cultural-sociological, not a legal, definition of the word "nation." No less than four car bombings were tied to militant separatists last year alone, and teams of heavily armed Canadian Mounties appear to have become a permanent fixture in Ottawa.

You occasionally think that the online photos of Canadian police give the appearance of storm troopers; but on the other hand, domestic terrorism to the north has gotten out of hand, and something must be done. Leaders of the Québécois movement disavowed the bombings, claiming that they were false-flag operations to demonize their cause, but few outside the movement believe that story. Some long-haul truckers from other provinces have joined the separatists, or at least wave the Québécois flag, though most don't speak a word of French. By 2024 their big rig trucks were all connected to the internet and the engine systems equipped with a kill switch that the government can deploy in emergencies. So the threat of the old trucker-convoy protests is long gone.

American society has gone entirely cashless—the old dollar bills, by now mostly removed from circulation, are no longer accepted anywhere and have already lost all value on the streets. A few remaining Luddites complain about the lack of tuckaway cash for the battered woman preparing to extricate herself from an abusive relationship, the impossibility of garage sales or cash donations to the homeless person on the street corner. Grandparents neither discreetly slip cash into their grandchild's hand nor slip money into birthday cards. Street performers don't put out hats for tips. Children's piggy banks are useless, and the tooth fairy no longer visits.

But the city's homeless don't beg for money anyways. Seattle finally solved its out-of-control homeless problem when officials discovered that most of the city's homeless population did not want housing, but were content and pacified when provided tents, food, virtual reality, and the new synthetic cannabinoid-opioid-benzodiazepine formulation, Reverie. The new drug comes in a pill that easily dissolves under the tongue, doing away with the needle-exchange programs that social conservatives complained about. Washington legalized Reverie in 2027, and the drug is mass produced cheaply at a facility in Walla Walla.

At first, homeless individuals with schizophrenia sometimes inadvertently broke the VR sets provided by the city, but higher doses of Reverie solved most of that by calming their intermittent agitation. For the remainder of the mentally ill homeless—in a government program that actually worked—Seattle partnered with a military contractor that provided industrial-grade VR sets that were "Virtually Unbreakable," according to their marketing tagline. The homeless no longer bothered anyone and rarely crapped on the sidewalks downtown anymore, having decamped to nearby Ballard, where free Reverie, VR, and heavy-duty tents were provided with funding from King County. High school dropouts often took the bus there to hang out with the homeless and partake of the R&F, as they called it: Reverie & Fantasy. Some of these ended up permanently opting for the R&F lifestyle.

Reverie now comes in nine different personalized, color-coded versions, formulated to match the most common genomic and EEG brain profiles. According to your Health app algorithm, you respond best to Blue Reverie, though Orange Reverie may be necessary when you're especially stressed. But you've generally stayed away from the drug: Reverie tends to be frowned upon by your employer, Microsoft, where management has expressed concerns the drug may slow employee productivity.

Your company health plan does, however, provide free access to Keen, Pfizer's new cognitive enhancer approved by the FDA last year, which is similarly available in six personalized color-coded variations. Your gene sequence and EEG profile indicate that Green Keen will help you get going in the morning, especially after a night of suboptimal sleep. Most days you don't feel you need it, so you stick with old-fashioned espresso—still a Seattle staple.

Everyone in the United States now has a digital ID. As of five years ago, DMVs only issue digital driver's licenses, and paper passports were phased out four years ago. You cannot deny the conveniences of this advance: your digital ID contains all your medical records and emergency information, easily available to you and accessible to your doctors or the EMTs arriving on the scene should you suffer an unfortunate fall or accident. This came in handy last year when you went over the handlebars of your mountain bike and broke your collarbone. With the new medical enhancements, you sometimes forget you're forty-five and probably shouldn't be hitting the jumps on the biking trail. Obtaining routine health care requires fewer visits to a physician, given the new biometrics-AI system that interfaces with your Health app.

Your wearable biometric ring sends data to your smartphone, providing moment-to-moment monitoring of your heart-rate-variability, phases of sleep, body temperature, skin conductance, and blood oxygenation. The new waterproof version does not need to be removed in the shower, so it stays permanently on the ring finger of your right hand, complementing the wedding ring on your left. The bio-ring contracts occasionally, gently squeezing your finger to take your blood pressure. You get a monthly reminder on your phone for a pinprick blood sample, which can be done at home on a small device that also interfaces with your smartphone. You are prompted quarterly to pee on a stick, which you insert into the same home-testing device.

Your biometric ring is something of an anachronism. Friends chide you about still wearing it and ridicule the crude metrics it delivers. Like most people, they converted over a year ago to an implantable nanotechnology device. This device communicates with a barely visible graphene bioimpedance tattoo[3] placed on the skin just over the radial artery to measure blood pressure and skin conductance. "You're still using VHS in a world of Blu-ray and HD streaming," your coworker tells you. For some reason, you just can't get past your idiosyncratic hang-up about implanting the half-centimeter cylinder under the skin. "Would you refuse a pacemaker for your heart, Mr. Dinosaur?" your best friend teases. Maybe next year I'll get it done, you think.

You do appreciate that all your medications are now nanotechnology-enabled: each pill contains a tiny seed that sends an electronic signal to your Health app once the pill dissolves in your stomach.[4] Now, if you forget whether you took the pill that morning, you can verify on your phone. Doctors and health insurance companies also appreciate being able to monitor medication compliance for their patients and clients.

Almost everyone wears glasses, though not to improve their vision. Most of your friends have converted their smartphone to elegant-looking smart glasses that interface with their subcutaneous biometric ID chip or bio-ring. You've ordered yours, but supply chain problems have delayed delivery (there were too many lockdowns in 2028, again). Your neighbor explains that while she used to always forget her phone—it was too bulky for her pocket, and she'd never been good at keeping track of her purse—her new Ray-Ban smart glasses conveniently stay on her face. Plus, if you don't want to use the glasses' lenses as your screen (which are admittedly not quite as good as the best smartphones), or if the glasses battery runs out, most venues have larger universal screens where you can easily access your personalized data with a facial ID or fingerprint.

Your big-data Health app's algorithm, funded by the NIH and run by private firms, analyzes your biometric information in real time, combining it with your sequenced genome, structural and functional body scans, and family history automatically linked from your family members' Health app profiles. You receive weekly reports in your inbox and notifications on your phone regarding your sleep metrics, stress level, exercise, and diet, along with recommendations for medications and other products that might improve your health profile and lower your risk of various diseases.

The "ask your doctor about" commercials on your social media feed are now remarkably individualized, addressing you by name and explaining the benefits of the personalized recommendations. With changes to FDA regulations, many of the advertised products no longer require a prescription: the Health app algorithm can make most diagnoses and treatment recommendations independently. Consequently, accessing health care requires far fewer physician visits than a few years ago. Societal safety has also improved with biometric surveillance: drunk driving fatalities are way down since most cars are self-driving. The manual cars are impossible to start if the algorithm detects that your blood alcohol level is over the legal limit.

Advances in design and functionality made N99 masks required at virtually all public gatherings during flu and covid seasons up until last year. There were still a few mask dissidents around—the folks who rarely go out for several months a year—but most people agreed that it's best to mask up and keep everyone safe. New variants of covid and influenza often escape vaccine immunity, a problem that continues to plague vaccine research. Last year, mask mandates were dropped when the city of Seattle began implementing its facial ID safety and surveillance system downtown. Masks were a hindrance to the system's smooth functioning. In the first year of the facial ID system's coming online, crime rates from petty theft and vandalism finally dropped in Seattle after having risen for several previous years.

You are a bit uncomfortable that your biometric ring–enabled Health app, by analyzing your vital signs and bodily movements while you are in bed, seems to know that you have recently developed situational erectile dysfunction and that physical intimacy with your wife has declined. Your social media feeds now have a flood of ads for Fulsome, Johnson & Johnson's new erectile dysfunction medication. But for the most part, you appreciate the ability to easily monitor your health and fine-tune your diet, physical activity, and medication regimen without inconvenient trips to the doctor's office.

When you need to see the doc, telemedicine has replaced almost all in-person visits. Thank goodness, your annual rectal exam to monitor prostate health is a thing of the past (the biometric algorithm does a better job). You read in the paper this morning that colonoscopies will also soon be phased out, about which you are not complaining. Nor is your wife complaining that they are now saying the same thing about mammograms.

As part of a subscription program, you receive a package in the mail twice a year with personalized DNA/mRNA vials, which you can either self-inject at home or bring to a local pharmacy for administration if you are squeamish about needles. The instructional video on your Health app was all you needed to get comfortable giving yourself the shots. One injection you took last year increased your muscle mass by 8 percent without any changes to your workout routine. A coworker claims she found an enhancement that boosted her cognition even more effectively than Keen. She credits the shot for improving her bridge game and increasing her productivity at work. "I'm spending 14 percent less time on programming, according to my Work app," she tells you one day at the watercooler. "You've got to try this one." You jot down the name of the product. Progress is good.

While you can still buy on credit, the old plastic credit cards are no longer used, and your eight-year-old daughter has never heard of writing a check. You are happy that you don't need to remember logins or passwords for dozens of online accounts anymore because your digital ID ties into everything. A quick iris scan logs you into all your accounts, allows you to make purchases, and gets you admittance to any venue where you've purchased a ticket. With these scans, combined with Index of Social Responsibility (ISR) scores, security lines at the airport move much faster than they did five years ago.

Thanks to the Americans with Disabilities Act, facial ID is available at all venues for those with corneal cataracts or other eye problems that might impair iris scans. You still use your iPhone 16, though you don't need to swipe QR codes or use Apple Pay anymore. So the phone spends more time in your pocket while you're on the go. It's not much of a hassle if you forget your phone at home, even when going to the airport—your iris scan will do just fine for almost everything, including a boarding pass and digital ID—which saved you on your last trip from Seattle to San Francisco.

● ● ●

Notwithstanding these conveniences and advances, you do notice some flies in the ointment. Your nephew Jordan hit a rough patch at age nineteen, got hooked on methamphetamine, and was caught by police selling the drug to support his own habit—a felony. He did some jail time, found God in prison, completed a Twelve Step recovery program, and has remained clean, sober, and on the straight and narrow for the past two years since his release. Jordan hopes someday to settle down and start a family. But he has been consistently unable to find a job or even land an interview since he got out of prison. Although he is ready to work, his life has completely stalled. He's quite convinced that taking online courses for his associate's degree will not improve his employment prospects.

Although Jordan paid his debt to society and straightened out his life, private companies still have access to his criminal, drug use, and financial history. Even with purported legal privacy protections on some of this information and laws intended to protect him from discrimination, corporations readily glean sufficient data from other social credit indices to put the pieces together and reconstruct his history with near certainty. Where else but jail would one be unable to make a single purchase for several years? His pattern of movements in specific neighborhoods just before that gap in market transactions, combined with biometric measures indicating the abuse of stimulants during that period, confirm a history of methamphetamine and/or cocaine addiction with 99.2 percent certainty.

While your nephew receives a universal-basic-income digital deposit from the Federal Reserve each month, his actual purchasing power is limited, so most of those modest funds stay parked in his digital bank account. The government encourages him to spend the money on education or green transportation, but there are other things he would like to do with the funds. He can still shop at Costco and Walmart, but his personalized digital dollar is no good at Whole Foods and Macy's, and certainly not at Nordstrom or Saks. Even if he wins the lottery, his ISR score will never be high enough for him to stay at the Four Seasons.

Jordan still can't get a reservation at most restaurants in the city, much less a ticket to the Seattle Symphony or Fifth Avenue and Paramount Theaters. Movie theaters only issue him tickets to the matinee times unless he is willing to pay double (an ISR score adjustment fee), so it's been hard to take any woman he meets on a decent date. His housing options are likewise extremely limited, as he quickly learns whenever he tries to rent an apartment. Because of these roadblocks, your nephew recently moved back home with your brother and sister-in-law, even though he could afford to live on his own. That pretty much put the nail in the coffin on his prospects for finding a decent woman to marry: most were not interested in watching immersive movies or sports in his parents' basement VR room. Jordan is now feeling quite stuck and demoralized. You worry that he'll relapse on meth or take up the R&F lifestyle with the Ballard bums.

Your ISR score—the Index of Social Responsibility metric is the one Washington State has adopted, though there are several other versions—is such that you don't encounter the same kinds of difficulties as Jordan. However, you are almost convinced that your political leanings and charitable donations sometimes result in deprioritization in competitive market transactions, limit access to some special perks your friends qualify for, and may have created a permanent glass ceiling at work. But these hunches are impossible to prove. Though you don't like to admit it to yourself, you probably do monitor more carefully what news stories you click on and what websites you visit.

You advise your children to be extremely careful about what they purchase, watch, and listen to, and to be mindful about where they go, whom they associate with online or in person, and what they like or whom they follow on social media. If they are not scrupulous about these things, their college admission prospects could be compromised. Again, you cannot prove this, but everyone now knows it's true. Three years ago, your children accused you of being paranoid when you gave this kind of advice; but now they and their friends all understand this and stringently police their own behavior.

Last year saw a round of international climate lockdowns—now termed RRPs—Rejuvenation & Reprieve Periods—which Seattle enthusiastically embraced. However, these RRPs came on the heels of the annual covid-season lockdown, the combination of which provoked citywide riots in nearby Tacoma. This city to the south, long known as the "armpit of Seattle," had inadequate public transportation options for blue-collar workers who could not work from home. Workers' cars, all connected to the internet, would not start during the last RRP unless their biometric data indicated they were experiencing a health emergency and needed to go to the hospital.

Since the trouble in Tacoma, most people now avoid driving south of Seattle on the Interstate 5, unless they need to go to Sea-Tac airport. Everett's new airport, north of the city, has plans to expand and will likely become the new international hub. Tacoma and the surrounding areas still look like a charred wasteland, and the city is having difficulty hiring police and firefighters, much less cleanup crews. The residents who could afford to leave have already fled Tacoma, most of them moving to Montana to find work in the recently discovered lithium mines near Bozeman. New cars are required to run on batteries, and gas stations are closing down as the old cars from the "gasoline age" fade from the scene. Other Tacoma residents made their way to the Walla Walla Reverie factory looking for work. A few have stayed, but the city looks like a burned-out ghost town.

Rumors have it that a group of dissident anarchists are squatting in the old Tacoma Dome, but police won't go near it and most people dismiss the rumors as urban legend. Other rumors suggest that civil unrest is a growing problem elsewhere around the country, although those who don't travel much outside the big cities dismiss this possibility because they never see anything about it on television or social media. "That's just populist propaganda," your brother tells you when you bring it up, so you don't mention it anymore at family gatherings. You often feel like it's become harder to know what's true or where to get accurate information.

The University of Washington in Seattle has emerged as the premier institution for the study of data science, and your division at Microsoft recruits heavily from UW. Washington State University in Pullman is known for its tech, pharmaceutical science, and manufacturing management degrees. As state funding is funneled to UW and WSU and their endowments grow from tech philanthropists, Western Washington University in Bellingham, a hundred miles north of Seattle, is slowly being starved of state funding and gets no major philanthropic gifts. Western still has a reputation for too many tenured "granola roller" faculty who reject ecomodernism in favor of old-school environmentalism, emphasizing small-scale local economies and resisting the global corporatization of the environmental movement.

Students at Western don Birkenstocks and "Small Is Beautiful" or "Dismantle the Megamachine" T-shirts while they study organic farming and read Rachel Carson and E. F. Schumacher. The early twentieth-century economic distributism theories of G. K. Chesterton and Hilaire Belloc are enjoying a revival among the campus's quirky Catholic subculture, and even among some Protestant students. The WWU student body and faculty still typically prefer natural marijuana to synthetic Reverie. History and philosophy have become popular majors among students, but of course funding for the humanities in higher education remains abysmal.

The old computer center at Western is home to several cranky dissident programmers who refuse to retire, complain endlessly about the loss of privacy, and rail against algorithmic governance. As funding declines, WWU student enrollment is down, and Bellingham's population has shrunk as university employees move to Seattle or Pullman. The city is home to many local cooperatives on the model of Preston, England's unorthodox "community wealth building" reform of 2012. But the co-ops now struggle with the decline of their customer base as residents move away. The ranks of Bellingham's dissident subcultures decline by the year.

The old St. Luke's Hospital in Bellingham, converted decades ago to a medical office building, now sits half-empty. The remaining tenants mostly consist of naturopaths and chiropractors who operate outside the "biopharmaceutical-industrial complex" and still dispense the old strains of natural medicinal cannabis rather than the new synthetic cannabinoids. They share office space with a couple of palliative-care physicians who remain licensed but whose board certification was revoked three years ago when they refused to euthanize their elderly patients with dementia. These are the only allopathic doctors in town who know why the building is still named for that "dear and glorious physician," the patron saint of medicine, and who have a copy of the Hippocratic Oath on their office wall.

In contrast to these marginalized critics of contemporary society, all the politicians and most of their constituents seem to agree that the national economy is booming and that Washington State represents the vanguard of progress, overtaking even California for that title. Pharmaceutical, medical device, and tech stocks are way up, as are stocks for the new data storage companies. Amazon Web Services now has two major competitors, as data has become the new oil. A few environmentalists complain that the enormous data storage facilities in Eastern Washington use more energy and have larger carbon footprints than the old gasoline cars, but most climate experts ignore them.

Drones deliver almost all goods, including food, from Amazon a guaranteed six hours after you order them online. Jeff Bezos is convinced he can bring that down to four hours in Seattle, if only the King County supervisors would agree to zoning changes permitting more local land for his warehouses. The company is also lobbying the city to subsidize better public transportation between the greater Seattle metro area and the other side of Steven's Pass. Aside from its executives and some of its upper management, none of Amazon's employees can afford to live on the west side of the Cascade Mountains.

As a software engineer at Microsoft who has moved up to an associate VP position, your standard of living has risen in the years since the covid pandemic. You now lease a Tesla SUV and minivan and time-share a new ski boat that you take out on Lake Washington in the summers. Your family regularly vacations in Europe in the summer on short-lease properties. You used to ski at Mount Baker, but these days you head to upscale Jackson Hole or Aspen for ski trips in the winter. Your stock portfolio is strong and leans heavily toward tech and the new big data companies.

Following successful trial runs in Bologna, Italy, in 2023, Seattle announced four years ago that, along with Palo Alto, San Jose, and San Francisco, it would become one of the first smart cities in the United States, incorporating "digital governance" principles into every aspect of civic life. The project promised to create "an ecosystem of public and private stakeholders serving citizens wherever they are." The city of Seattle recently contracted with Salesforce to create an integrated citizen-relationship management platform to upgrade its smart-city model. This announcement attracted even more tech-savvy young professionals to move to the region.

After the retirement of Marc Benioff, now a full-time consultant for the WEF, Peter Schwartz was promoted from senior vice president of strategic planning at Salesforce to the company's new CEO. Schwartz's bio describes him as "an internationally renowned futurist and business strategist, specializing in scenario planning and working with corporations, governments, and institutions to create alternative perspectives of the future."[5] Salesforce recently moved its headquarters to Bellevue, just across Lake Washington from Seattle, which has increased the value of your home in Seattle's University District even more since you purchased it twelve years ago.

Some conspiracy-types among the city's old bohemian crowd like to remind people that Peter Schwartz, Seattle's newest tech business mogul, previously maintained CIA connections and was the author of the Rockefeller-funded "Lock Step" pandemic-planning scenario back in 2009—a fictional war game that uncannily predicted the failed covid response. While the supposed document is cited in some old books, nobody can seem to find it on the internet. Most people in Seattle ignore these cranks and have embraced Schwartz, who bikes to work, recently made a multimillion-dollar gift to the Seattle Symphony, plans to fund a new city opera house, and has taken up mountaineering, hoping to climb Rainier next year—no small feat for a man his age.

Admittedly, traffic is terrible again with all the new transplants: they still have not built the promised subway system, and it's hard to construct more bridges across Seattle's lakes and Puget Sound. Traffic improved for a couple of years after the covid pandemic as more people continued to work from home, but the city's new transplants have led to congestion again. However, you work and shop from home almost exclusively, so you navigate city traffic only occasionally when you head downtown to attend Seahawks games. You've enjoyed season tickets through Microsoft for the last three years—the envy of your friends who don't happen to work in tech or finance.

Since you keep your carbon footprint and energy use low—you installed solar panels on your roof last year, even though the sky is grey nine months a year in Seattle—the city rewards your high ISR score with 20 percent off all concessions and parking at the football games, as well as discounted entrance to the Space Needle, the Seattle Science Center, and the Rock and Roll Museum downtown—a building whose architecture looks like a pile of laundry but is fun to visit when friends are in town. You also get discounts at Microsoft's cafeteria (not that you use it much working from home) as a company reward for being in the top quartile for your ISR. More satisfyingly, you won a $1,000 bet with a coworker in your division for beating him on the twelve-month ISR average last year. People at work have become remarkably competitive about the metric, ever since the company started posting everyone's score in a monthly team email.

But not everyone in Seattle appears to share in the bounty. You've met some of your nephew's friends, for example. Rates of free-floating anxiety and psychosomatic illnesses are sky-high. Everyone seems to have seasonal affective disorder, which requires periodic treatments. Chronic fatigue syndrome and idiopathic chronic pain have reached record levels, though new pharmaceutical drugs have mitigated some of the ill effects. You recently read that psychiatry has become an increasingly popular specialty among medical students at UW: demand for mental health care is way up, and the compensation in this field now rivals that for dermatology and orthopedics. Psychiatrists dispense not just conventional antipsychotics, anxiolytics, mood stabilizers, and antidepressants, but newer personalized drugs like cognitive enhancers and mood adjuvants.

Despite the economic gains and technological advances, everyone seems to know several people who have taken their own life in the years since the covid pandemic. The websites and marketing brochures at local private high schools like Bishop Blanchet and Seattle Prep boast not only impressive college admissions stats, but also highlight their ratio of one mental health counselor for every eighteen students. This has meant an increase in your kids' tuition bills, to be sure, but nobody among your friends or colleagues would dream of sending their kids to public schools, which are populated entirely by low-ISR families. Last year there were nine suicides at the local public high school, and even the private high schools continue to have several student suicides each year. Washington's governor, a former VP at Microsoft, has declared a "mental health pandemic" and pledged more public funding to address the problem.

Your anecdotal impression is that cancer is also up—an uncanny number of people you know seem to be on personalized chemotherapy regimens for blood cancers like leukemia and lymphoma. Chronic medical illness and unexplained autoimmune and neurological problems have also been on the rise, especially among those who can afford the routine DNA/mRNA regimens. In fact novel shots often seem to address problems that some people believe were exacerbated by prior shots. But again, it's hard to sift fact from fiction in these matters. Most people don't seem to care about epidemiology until one of these afflictions affects a loved one. People typically trust their Health app algorithm.

Most of the time, you feel healthier, though there was that bout two years ago where your hands when numb and tingly for ten weeks straight and your doctor couldn't explain it. He did prescribe a new drug for it, Neurontogen, which seemed to help. Eventually the mysterious symptoms remitted, except when your hands get too cold on the ski slopes. Your last mRNA shot improved not just your muscle mass but also your skiing endurance, so overall you're not complaining. The ten-year subscription of injections was on balance a good purchase.

· · ·

Your personal life hit a rough patch with your wife starting about six months ago. She struggles with seasonal affective disorder and chronic fatigue, and still has not found the right medication regimen. Your Work app algorithm has been keeping you working long hours to meet more demanding deadlines, and your productivity metrics have not recently been what they were a few years ago. You believe the stress at home is contributing to more distractions at work. After a recent argument with your wife, you noticed more ads on your social media and news feeds for Tindr and similar dating and hookup apps.

Last year, Washington, Oregon, California, and a dozen other states legalized health- and safety-approved erotic escort services. Biometric and location data now facilitates SSSW—Sanitary and Safe Sex Work—and the old-fashioned word "prostitution" has gone the way of "fornication." Tax revenues from these services, along with the heavily taxed Reverie, have generated welcome budget surpluses for the state this year. Blue-check-approved SSSW services are required by law to biometrically screen both their providers and clients for sexually transmitted infections, including ARG—antibiotic resistant gonorrhea, a very nasty bug that emerged in 2028 and nearly brought the sexual revolution to a grinding halt sixty years after it began. The screening guarantee provides clients added peace of mind and helps justify the higher price tag. Three blue-check approved SSSW companies in Seattle qualify for city subsidies, which allow the escorts to offer 60 percent discounts to the city's police and firefighters.

This finally resolved the Seattle Police Department's hiring headaches, which had plagued the city ever since the Capitol Hill Autonomous Zone (CHAZ) fiasco during the George Floyd protests of 2020. In what was not among the city's finest moments, with insufficient support from the mayor, Seattle police abandoned their East Precinct building, which was subsequently destroyed by the angry denizens of CHAZ. For several years afterwards, very few cops wanted to work for Seattle. But with the new SSSW escort perks, the city is now able to attract more than enough recruits, especially single men, to staff its police and fire departments. This development, combined with the new facial recognition camera system downtown, has boosted Seattle's safety and security: Seattle is now proudly ranked among the five safest cities in America.

SSSW escort services deploy highly refined personalized marketing to professionals, especially men who travel frequently. Professionals who purchase these services uniformly use the blue-check companies, even though unapproved services are considerably cheaper. In addition to the health screening functionality, the blue check guarantees that these transactions will not harm your ISR score. It is now clear from the ads on your social media feeds that SSSW services know your preferences for young, slender brunettes. While an increasing number of your colleagues at work avail themselves of these services while traveling, you reassured your worried wife that you never partake while on business trips.

However, after a major fight with her, you depart for a trip to San Francisco feeling lonely, misunderstood, and rejected. As you wait for your luggage at baggage claim, curiosity momentarily gets the best of you, and you impulsively click on one of the SSSW escort ads. Photos of five gorgeous, slender brunettes pop up. You hit the button on the most attractive one and within twelve seconds are connected via videoconferencing to the woman. She introduces herself as "Porsche, like the car," and asks, "Do you have any time before your meetings in Palo Alto tomorrow?"

"I, uh . . . I suppose," you mumble, wondering how she knows about your meeting plans at Stanford.

"Okay, I'll be outside baggage claim in ten minutes," she says, and hangs up before you have time to blink.

A notification for your "transportation service" immediately pops up telling you the make and model of the vehicle, a plug-in Escalade with plenty of room in the back seat. Clicking on the text message opens a discreet app that looks just like Uber and Lyft. You are already having second thoughts, but the service advertises that the transportation to your hotel is free of charge, and you figure you can always bail out after that.

The Escalade pulls up and you hesitate a moment before getting in the back seat. The woman turns out to be charming and very sweet, much more high-class than you imagined. In fact, Porsche looks and sounds remarkably like your favorite movie actress. She hands you a Blue

Reverie pill and your drink of choice. With advances in AI, most restaurant waitresses anticipate your order before you even look at the menu, so you're not surprised that Porsche knows that you prefer your eighteen-year single malt Macallan neat. You're feeling conflicted about this "transportation" plan, and your anxiety begins to rise, so you down the Reverie with a sip of scotch to calm your nerves.

It's not long before Porsche starts turning up the seductive temperature in the back seat of the Escalade. You pull back slightly from her initial advances and hesitate, but her personalized scents are delicious, her voice lovely, and her hand feels good on your knee. By the time you finish your drink, the car is only halfway to your Palo Alto hotel, and without fully realizing what is happening you find yourself enjoying the flirtation and giving in to the foreplay. You're also feeling the effects of the scotch and the Reverie—definitely a higher dose than you've tried in the past.

Your phone suddenly buzzes with a text from your eight-year-old daughter, interrupting the charged moment: "Do you know where my boots are?" Your brain snaps to, overcoming the buzzed sensations and the Reverie fog. Picturing your wife and kids, you suddenly wonder how you've allowed things to get this far. "I'm sorry," you mutter to Porsche, "it's not you . . . I, uh . . . I don't think I can do this." She is understanding and does not seem offended or put off. Her voice turns ever so slightly more businesslike but remains sweet: "You'll still be charged for the drink and 20 percent for cancellation, but it shows up on your bank statement as 'hotel transportation,'" she explains. You apparently forgot to read the fine print when you clicked "Agree" on the terms and conditions, but whatever.

As the Escalade pulls up to the hotel, you begin to wonder whether anyone who knows you might see you get out. After all, you have a lot of professional contacts in Silicon Valley. Without your asking, Porsche takes your hand to help you down from the SUV, gets out with you, and quickly plants a light kiss on your cheek before waving goodbye. "Text me through the app if you change your mind," she says. As the car drives away you look around, relieved that you don't recognize any familiar faces on the street. Three days later you arrive home from the trip sober, clear-headed, and committed to dialing back your work hours and focusing on rebuilding your marriage. You find the boots behind the sofa.

● ● ●

You are sitting at breakfast one morning the following month, reading Microsoft's weekly company update email as you sip your cappuccino. Your employer just announced that their DNA-programming research enterprise is moving from animal to human trials. As explained by Dr. Andrew Phillips, head of bio computation at Microsoft, back in 2016 when the project was in its infancy: "Imagine a biological computer that operates inside a living cell—for example, to determine if a cell is cancerous and then trigger the death of that cell."[6] The technology takes advantage of a process called DNA strand displacement, because as he explained, "DNA is highly programmable, just like a computer, and we can program a whole range of complex behaviors using DNA molecules." The potential biotechnology applications of Microsoft's proprietary software for programming molecular circuits made of DNA are limitless: "Ultimately it could allow us to make biological computers that operate at a molecular scale," Dr. Phillips maintains. Exciting news, you muse, pleased to be working for such a forward-looking enterprise.

You flick your screen to the *Seattle Times*. The first headline announces that London police are piloting the use of precog AI to anticipate and stop crimes before they happen—looks promising, you muse. A second headline catches your eye because it relates to your work: the article describes another major data-security breach in one of the large transnational data storage companies. Cybersecurity and intelligence experts believe the culprit is probably a major player somewhere outside the United States, perhaps even a foreign government. Data-security hacks like this have not exactly been rare occurrences over the past several years, so you don't give it much thought. Your professional expertise is not in privacy or encryption but in data compression and curation. So, unlike several of your colleagues, you won't be required to attend the emergency Teams sessions at work that day—for which you are not complaining.

These meetings are typically populated with a diverse group of foreign nationals cooperating in data-harm minimization. International law now mostly governs data privacy and protection regulations. This facilitates cooperation among citizens and regulatory consistency for multinational corporations like Microsoft, which now need fewer lawyers to navigate the numerous byzantine regulatory schemes in foreign countries. Ever since seven nations signed the Agile Nations Charter in November 2020,[7] dozens of other countries, including the United States, have also signed on, making the free flow of data, subject to uniform international regulations, the almost-universal norm globally. A few rogue nations have begun to harden their internet systems, contrary to these trends, and the concept of net neutrality remains hotly debated among policy wonks.

Agile Net advocates worry that if the internet regresses back to a collection of closed networks, the full potential of data sharing and AI will not be realized. But this seems unlikely, as most countries clearly agree on the benefits of a consistent worldwide regulatory system to govern the internet. Politicians from both parties encourage a culture of data sharing and open access among constituents. Agile Net's push for openness naturally requires enhanced AI algorithms to monitor online misinformation from foreign and domestic sources—nobody refers to information curation as censorship anymore. You recall how by 2024, we were swimming in a sea of such confusing information online that pretty much everyone—you included—agreed that the new streamlined systems of information flow are an advance over the old online cacophony.

Two days after reading about the latest data breach, you receive a phone call from one of the new interns at work, a Chinese graduate student working at Microsoft over the summer. He asks to meet you for coffee that day. You wonder if he might be interested in your work on big data compression or data curation. You're always keen to mentor the next generation in software programming, so you arrange to meet. The morning of the meeting, your brother calls you to lament that Jordan has relapsed on meth, which puts you in a dyspeptic mood. You're hoping that an opportunity to advise a young programmer with a bright future might help set things right. However, moments after you sit down with him at the local Starbucks you sense that something is off with this guy.

He tells you he needs your cooperation at work to gain a back door into a data-curation algorithm you're working on. You blink, squint at him, then stare down at your cappuccino, confused, and wonder if you heard him correctly—his English is admittedly not great. Just then, he takes out his smartphone and plays for you an audio recording. You recognize your own voice on the recording as well as . . . what was her name? . . . Porsche's voice. It dawns on you that this is your conversation in the backseat of the Escalade. The intern scrubs ahead on the recording, and you can hear the sound of her dirty talk and your kissing.

The intern flicks his screen again and shows you the de-encrypted transaction fee you paid to the escort company, followed by a photo of Porsche leaning into your ear with a goodbye kiss when you got out of the car. The photo was evidently taken from one of the many facial recognition towers that dot the streets of Palo Alto like old telephone poles. "I have also your browsing history," the intern tells you, "and a lot more." You rack your brain trying to think of what else he might have on you. But clearly the tryst with the escort is more than enough.

"You are going to help me," the intern says again in a matter-of-fact monotone voice. "I need your iris scan to access the system. You do not want your wife and kids to receive anything from me in their inboxes tomorrow." You wonder whether your wife would believe you if you explained that you interrupted the escort encounter early, but it's no use. Even if she does believe you, things quite obviously still went too far. There will be no explaining it to her, much less to the kids.

"What is the line the old book say," your young adversary asks in his imperfect English, "Big Brother always watching?" You stare dumbstruck at his self-satisfied wry grin. Yes, you've read Orwell, but for crying out loud this is not *Nineteen Eighty-Four*; this is not some sci-fi dystopian fantasy! This is your real life. This is Seattle, 2030.

You suddenly break into a cold sweat, your mouth goes dry, and you feel lightheaded and a bit short of breath. Noting your sudden shift in vital signs and skin conduction, your Health app algorithm registers your extreme stress level. Siri's voice on your iPhone interrupts the conversation:

> You are likely experiencing a panic attack. Lorazepam is available at the CVS across the street—your diagnostic and prescription codes have been shared with all nearby pharmacies. You may also need a medical evaluation to rule-out a heart attack. Chest pain radiating down the left arm is a characteristic symptom of cardiac arrest. Say "yes" if you are experiencing any chest pain. The nearest emergency room is Harborview Medical Center, three miles away. Say "hospital" if you would like me to summon an ambulance . . .

Notes

Prologue: Nuremberg, 1947

1. Francis Galton, "Eugenics, Its Definition, Scope, and Aims," *American Journal of Sociology* 10, no. 1 (1904): 5.
2. Samantha Young, "California Lawmakers Seek Reparations for People Sterilized by the State," *Washington Post*, April 25, 2018, https://www.washingtonpost.com/national /health-science/california-lawmakers-seek-reparations-for-people-sterilized-by-the-state /2018/04/25/2a873578-4869-11e8-8082-105a446d19b8_story.html.
3. "Laughlin's Model Law," Harry Laughlin and Eugenics, 2020, https://historyofeugenics .truman.edu/altering-lives/sterilization/model-law/.
4. Cited in Andrea Patterson, "Germs and Jim Crow: The Impact of Microbiology on Public Health Policies in Progressive Era American South," *Journal of the History of Biology* 42, no. 3 (Fall 2009): 529–59, http://users.clas.ufl.edu/davidson/Jim%20Crow%20America %20Spring%202016/Jim%20Crow%20America%20course%20readings/week%2011 %20Health,%20Life%20and%20Death/Patterson%202009.pdf.
5. Cf. Thomas C. Leonard, *Illiberal Reformers: Race, Eugenics, and American Economics in the Progressive Era* (Princeton: Princeton University Press, 2017).
6. Steve Usdin, "New Documents Reveal FDR's Eugenic Project to 'Resettle' Jews during World War II," Tablet, April 29, 2018, https://www.tabletmag.com/sections/arts-letters/ articles/m-project-franklin-delano-roosevelt-jews.
7. *Buck v. Bell*, 274 U.S. 200 (1927), https://supreme.justia.com/cases/federal/us/274/200/.
8. Bleecker Van Wagenen, *Preliminary Report of the Committee of the Eugenic Section of the American Breeder's Association to Study and to Report on the Best Practical Means for Cutting off the Defective Germ-Plasm in the Human Population* (Adelphi, Wisconsin: The Eugenics Education Society, 1912), https://readingroom.law.gsu.edu/cgi/viewcontent .cgi?article=1073&context=buckvbell.
9. Edwin Black, "Hitler's Debt to America," *The Guardian*, February 5, 2004, https://www .theguardian.com/uk/2004/feb/06/race.usa.
10. Robert N. Proctor, *Racial Hygiene: Medicine under the Nazis* (Cambridge, Massachusetts: Harvard University Press, 1988), 95–117.
11. Ibid.

12. Nuremberg Code, from *Trials of War Criminals before the Nuernberg Military Tribunals under Control Council Law No. 10. Nuernberg, October 1946–April 1949*, vol. 2 (Washington, D.C.: U.S. Government Printing Office, 1949), 181–82.

13. Jess Craig, "The Controversial Quest to Make a 'Contagious' Vaccine," *National Geographic*, March 18, 2022, https://www.nationalgeographic.com/science/article/the -controversial-quest-to-make-a-contagious-vaccine.

14. Pat Hagan, "The Vaccine That Spreads Immunity by Passing Itself On like a Virus," *Daily Mail*, February 21, 2022, https://www.dailymail.co.uk/health/article-10536697 /The-vaccine-spreads-immunity-passing-like-virus.html.

15. Ibid.

16. Ibid.

Chapter 1: Locked Up: The Biomedical Security State

1.   Katherine Fung, "Banks Have Begun Freezing Accounts Linked to Trucker Protest," *Newsweek*, February 18, 2022, https://www.newsweek.com/banks-have-begun-freezing -accounts-linked-trucker-protest-1680649.

2.   Peter Shawn Taylor, "Frozen: How Canada's Banks Betrayed Their Customers during the Emergencies Act," *C2C Journal*, May 4, 2022, https://c2cjournal.ca/2022/05/frozen-how -canadas-banks-betrayed-their-customers-during-the-emergencies-act/.

3.   Canadian Civil Liberties Association (@cancivlib), "The federal government has not met . . . ," Twitter, February 14, 2022, 7:36 p.m., https://twitter.com/cancivlib/status /1493383579983917057?s=20&t=ZmFKBeKEE6ZkRBq1lnSNoA.

4.   Douglas Farrow, "Complacency and Complicity: A Rejoinder by Douglas Farrow," Theopolis Institute, March 10, 2022, https://theopolisinstitute.com/conversations /complacency-and-complicity-a-rejoinder-by-douglas-farrow%EF%BF%BC%EF%BF %BC/.

5.   "Summary of Terrorism Threat to the U.S. Homeland," Department of Homeland Security, February 7, 2022, https://www.dhs.gov/ntas/advisory/national-terrorism -advisory-system-bulletin-february-07-2022. The bulletin included the following: "Key factors contributing to the current heightened threat environment include . . . the proliferation of false or misleading narratives, which sow discord or undermine public trust in U.S. government institutions: For example, there is widespread online proliferation of false or misleading narratives regarding . . . COVID-19. Grievances associated with these themes inspired violent extremist attacks during 2021. . . . As COVID-19 restrictions continue to decrease nationwide, increased access to commercial and government facilities and the rising number of mass gatherings could provide increased opportunities for individuals looking to commit acts of violence to do so, often with little or no warning. Meanwhile, COVID-19 mitigation measures—particularly COVID-19 vaccine and mask mandates—have been used by domestic violent extremists to justify violence since 2020 and could continue to inspire these extremists to target government, healthcare, and academic institutions that they associate with those measures." The bulletin cites no actual incidents of such violence, likely because there were none to cite.

6.   Nina Jankowicz et al., "Malign Creativity: How Gender, Sex, and Lies Are Weaponized against Women Online," Wilson Center, 2021, https://www.wilsoncenter.org/publication /malign-creativity-how-gender-sex-and-lies-are-weaponized-against-women-online.

7.   Nina Jankowicz (@wiczipedia), "The biggest challenge in identifying this content . . . ," Twitter, January 25, 2021, 10:10 a.m., https://twitter.com/wiczipedia/status /1353722007138009088.

8.   Nina Jankowicz (@wiczipedia), "Trump speech is definitely the most presidential thing he's ever done . . . ," Twitter, January 13, 2021, 6:32 p.m., https://twitter.com/wiczipedia /status/1349499639452594181.

9.   el gato malo, "the disinformation governance board would be the american 'ministry of truth,'" bad cattitude (Substack), April 27, 2022, https://boriquagato.substack.com/p/the -disinformation-governance-board.

10. Gerald F. Seib, "In Crisis, Opportunity for Obama," *Wall Street Journal*, November 21, 2008, https://www.wsj.com/articles/SB122721278056345271; Stewart D. Friedman, "Do

Not Waste This Crisis," *Harvard Business Review*, November 25, 2008, https://hbr.org/2008/11/dont-waste-this-crisis.

11. Giorgio Agamben, *Where Are We Now?: The Epidemic as Politics* (Lanham, Maryland: Rowman & Littlefield, 2021).

12. Luke Kemp, "The 'Stomp Reflex': When Governments Abuse Emergency Powers," BBC Future, April 28, 2021, https://www.bbc.com/future/article/20210427-the-stomp-reflex-when-governments-abuse-emergency-powers.

13. Agamben, *Where Are We Now?*, 9.

14. The concept and basic features of the biosecurity model were sketched back in 2013 by Patrick Zylberman, professor of the history of health in Paris, in an important book called "Microbial Storms." *Tempêtes microbiennes. Essai sur la politique de sécurité sanitaire dans le monde transatlantique* (Paris: Gallimard, 2013). Zylberman's account of these civic duty campaigns is found on pages 401–3, 425. While this book is not yet available in English, I am working with benefactors to publish an English translation of this book as well as Zylberman's brief book on the covid pandemic, "Forgetting Wuhan." Zylberman's work on biosecurity is foundational.

15. Cited in Russell A. Berman, "State of Emergency," *First Things*, no. 324 (June/July 2022), 19–25, https://www.firstthings.com/article/2022/06/state-of-emergency.

16. Ibid.

17. Ibid.

18. Giorgio Agamben, "Biosecurity and Politics," Strategic Culture Foundation, June 2, 2020, https://www.strategic-culture.org/news/2020/06/02/biosecurity-and-politics/; Deidre McPhillips, "Gates Foundation Donations to WHO Nearly Match Those from U.S. Government," *U.S. News & World Report*, May 29, 2020, https://www.usnews.com/news/articles/2020-05-29/gates-foundation-donations-to-who-nearly-match-those-from-us-government.

19. Pepe Escobar, "How Biosecurity Is Enabling Digital Neo-Feudalism," Strategic Culture Foundation, May 15, 2020, https://www.strategic-culture.org/news/2020/05/15/how-biosecurity-is-enabling-digital-neo-feudalism/.

20. Zylberman, *Tempêtes microbiennes*.

21. Agamben, "Biosecurity and Politics."

22. Lydia Ramsey Pflanzer, "A Report That Helped Convince Trump to Take Coronavirus Seriously Projected That 2.2 Million People Could Die in the US If We Don't Act," Business Insider, March 17, 2020, https://www.businessinsider.com/coronavirus-uk-report-projects-2-million-deaths-without-action-2020-3?op=1.

23. Agamben, "Biosecurity and Politics."

24. Ibid.

25. Escobar, "How Biosecurity Is Enabling Digital Neo-Feudalism."

26. Berman, "State of Emergency."

27. Brennan Center for Justice, *A Guide to Emergency Powers and Their Use* (New York: Brennan Center for Justice, 2019), https://www.brennancenter.org/media/4976/download.

28. Zylberman, *Tempêtes microbiennes*, 445. Cf. "Zylberman's Biosecurity Strategy Studies," The Indomitable Neoliberals FC, February 17, 2021, https://corpcoinc.wordpress.com/2021/02/17/zylbermans-biosecurity-strategy-studies/.

29. Alex Gutentag, "The Great Covid Class War," The Bellows, December 16, 2020, https://www.thebellows.org/the-great-covid-class-war/.

30. Michael Tracey, "Academia Is Establishing a Permanent Surveillance Bureaucracy That Will Soon Govern the Rest of the Country," Michael Tracy (Substack), September 21, 2021, https://mtracey.substack.com/p/academia-is-establishing-a-permanent.

31. Ibid.

32. Ibid.

33. Ibid.

34. Ibid.

35. Ibid.

36. Michael Tracey (@mtracey), "98% of students and faculty at Georgetown are vaccinated . . . ," Twitter, September 14, 2021, 9:50 p.m., https://twitter.com/mtracey/status/1437957019055579137.

37. Michael Tracey (@mtracey), "At USC Law School, the Dean has repeatedly urged students to confront and report on 'community members . . . ,'" Twitter, September 20, 2021, 8:12 p.m., https://twitter.com/mtracey/status/1440106732223705088.

38. Jay Greene, "Amazon's Employee Surveillance Fuels Unionization Efforts: 'It's Not Prison, It's Work,'" *Washington Post*, December 2, 2021, https://www.washingtonpost.com/technology/2021/12/02/amazon-workplace-monitoring-unions/.

39. Ibid.

40. Ibid.

41. Ibid.

42. Cf. Eugene McCarraher, *The Enchantments of Mammon: How Capitalism Became the Religion of Modernity* (Cambridge, Massachussetts: Harvard Belknap Press, 2019), 650.

43. Lauren Aratani, "Robots on the Rise as Americans Experience Record Job Losses amid Pandemic," *The Guardian*, February 27, 2020, https://www.theguardian.com/technology/2020/nov/27/robots-replacing-jobs-automation-unemployment-us.

44. Cf. McCarraher, *Enchantments of Mammon*, 482.

45. World Economic Forum, *The Future of Jobs Report* (Geneva: World Economic Forum, 2020), https://www.weforum.org/reports/the-future-of-jobs-report-2020.

46. Greene, "Amazon's Employee Surveillance."

47. Paul Kingsnorth, "Chasing the Dragon: Thoughts on St George's Day," The Abbey of Misrule (Substack), April 23, 2022, https://paulkingsnorth.substack.com/p/chasing-the-dragon.

48. Brackets in the original. Jay Greene and Chris Alcantara, "Amazon Warehouse Workers Suffer Serious Injuries at Higher Rates Than Other Firms," *Washington Post*, June 1, 2021, https://www.washingtonpost.com/technology/2021/06/01/amazon-osha-injury-rate.

49. "Do Not Allow Jeff Bezos to Return to Earth," Change.org, https://www.change.org/p/the-proletariat-do-not-allow-jeff-bezos-to-return-to-earth.

50. Emily Kirkpatrick, "There's Now a Guillotine Set Up Outside Jeff Bezos's Mansion," *Vanity Fair*, August 28, 2020, https://www.vanityfair.com/style/2020/08/jeff-bezos-guillotine-protest-amazon-workers.

51. I owe these anecdotes to Paul Kingsnorth, who writes about the machine in, among other Substack articles in the series, "A Thousand Mozarts," The Abbey of Misrule (Substack), July 3, 2021, https://paulkingsnorth.substack.com/p/a-thousand-mozarts?s=r.

52. Cited in Paul Kingsnorth, "Blanched Sun, Blinded Man," The Abbey of Misrule (Substack), May 26, 2021, https://paulkingsnorth.substack.com/p/blanched-sun-blinded-man?s=r.

53. Ibid.

54. Ibid.

55. Ibid.

56. Patrick Kingsly, "Israel's Spy Agency Will Track Omicron Patients' Phones, at Least through Thursday," *New York Times*, November 29, 2021, https://www.nytimes.com/live/2021/11/29/world/omicron-variant-covid/israel-covid-phone-tracking.

57. Noé Chartier, "Gov't Can't Be Trusted with Cellphone Tracking amid Pandemic: Former Ontario Privacy Commissioner," *Epoch Times*, December 29, 2021, https://www.theepochtimes.com/govt-cant-be-trusted-with-cellphone-tracking-amid-pandemic-former-ontario-privacy-commissioner_4182404.html.

58. Joseph Cox, "CDC Tracked Millions of Phones to See If Americans Followed COVID Lockdown Orders," *Vice*, May 3, 2022, https://www.vice.com/en/article/m7vymn/cdc-tracked-phones-location-data-curfews.

59. Yves-Alexandre de Montjoye et al., "Unique in the Crowd: The Privacy Bounds of Human Mobility," *Scientific Reports* 3, no. 1376 (2013): 1–5, https://doi.org/10.1038/srep01376.

60. Cox, "CDC Tracked Millions."

61. ACLU (@ACLU), "BREAKING: Newly declassified documents reveal that the CIA has been secretly conducting massive surveillance programs . . . ," Twitter, February 10, 2022, 7:51 p.m., https://twitter.com/ACLU/status/1491937850887180288.

62. Ron Wyden and Martin Heinrich, letter to Avril D. Haines and William J. Burns, April 13, 2021, https://www.wyden.senate.gov/imo/media/doc/HainesBurns_WydenHeinrich_13APR21%20-FINAL.pdf; "Wyden and Heinrich: Newly Declassified Documents Reveal Previously Secret CIA Bulk Collection, Problems with CIA Handling of Americans' Information," Ron Wyden: United States Senator for Oregon, February 10, 2022, https://www.wyden.senate.gov/news/press-releases/wyden-and-heinrich-newly -declassified-documents-reveal-previously-secret-cia-bulk-collection-problems-with-cia -handling-of-americans-information.

63. Ross Anderson, "The Panopticon Is Already Here," *The Atlantic*, September 20, 2020, https://www.theatlantic.com/magazine/archive/2020/09/china-ai-surveillance/614197/.

64. Jeremy Weissman, *The Crowdsourced Panopticon: Conformity and Control on Social Media* (Lanham, Maryland: Rowman & Littlefield, 2021), 39.

65. Jeremy Bentham, *Panopticon* (London: T. Payne, 1791).

66. George Orwell, *Nineteen Eighty-Four* (London: Secker and Warburg, 1949), 1–2.

67. Quoted in Taylor Dotson, "The Twitter Surveillance State," *New Atlantis* 79 (Winter 2022), https://www.thenewatlantis.com/publications/the-twitter-surveillance-state.

68. Ibid.

69. Ibid.

70. D. T. Max, "The Public-Shaming Pandemic," *New Yorker*, September 28, 2020, https://www.newyorker.com/magazine/2020/09/28/the-public-shaming-pandemic.

71. Ibid.

72. Zylberman, *Tempêtes microbiennes*, 405.

73. Robert F. Kennedy Jr., *The Real Anthony Fauci: Bill Gates, Big Pharma, and the Global War on Democracy and Public Health* (New York: Skyhorse, 2021), 382.

74. Ibid.

75. centerforhealthsecurity, "Event 201 Pandemic Exercise: Highlights Reel," YouTube, November 4, 2019, https://www.youtube.com/watch?v=AoLw-Q8X174&list= PL9-oVXQX88esnrdhaiuRdXGG7XOVYB9Xm.

76. Ibid.

77. Rockefeller Foundation and Global Business Network, *Scenarios for the Future of Technology and International Development* (New York: Rockefeller Foundation, 2010), 18, https://www.unapcict.org/resources/ictd-infobank/scenarios-future-technology-and -international-development.

78. Ibid., 19.

79. Ibid., 19, 21.

80. "NTI I Bio, Munich Security Conference Convene Global Leaders for Annual Tabletop Exercise on Reducing High-Consequence Biological Threats," NTI, March 18, 2021, https://www.nti.org/news/nti-bio-munich-security-conference-convene-global-leaders -annual-tabletop-exercise-reducing-high-consequence-biological-threats/.

81. Chris Morris, "U.S. Government Places $119 million Order for 13 Million Freeze-Dried Monkeypox Vaccines," *Fortune*, May 19, 2020, https://fortune.com/2022/05/19/ monkeypox-vaccine-purchase-2022-us-government/.

82. Robert W. Malone, "Monkey Pox: Truth versus Fearporn," Who Is Robert Malone (Substack), May 21, 2022, https://rwmalonemd.substack.com/p/monkey-pox; Caden Pearson, "California, Illinois Join New York to Declare Monkeypox States of Emergency," *Epoch Times*, August 1, 2022, https://www.theepochtimes.com/illinois -california-governors-declare-monkeypox-states-of-emergency_4636793.html.

83. Zylberman, *Tempêtes microbiennes*; cf. also: Committee on Government Reform, *One Year Later: Evaluating the Effectiveness of Project BioShield, Hearing before the Committee on Government Reform, House of Representatives* (Washington, D.C.: U.S. Government Printing Office, 2005), https://www.govinfo.gov/content/pkg/CHRG -109hhrg23143/pdf/CHRG-109hhrg23143.pdf.

84. WEF, "A Cyber Attack with COVID Like Characteristics," YouTube, March 29, 2021, https://www.youtube.com/watch?v=Gm-7mcR86QU.

85. Wikipedia, s.v. "Article 48 (Weimar Constitution)," May 29, 2022, https://en.wikipedia.org/wiki/Article_48_(Weimar_Constitution).

86. Kemp, "The 'Stomp Reflex.'"
87. Daniel Spencer and Panetta McGrath, "12 Commandments to Avoid AHPRA Notifications," MIPS, February 28, 2022, https://support.mips.com.au/home/12-commandments-to-avoid-ahpra-notifications.
88. "Professional Expectations regarding Medical Misinformation and Disinformation," FSMB, April 2022, https://www.fsmb.org/siteassets/advocacy/policies/ethics-committee-report-misinformation-april-2022-final.pdf; Kylee Griswold, "Top Medical Licensure Board Creates Misinformation Policy—Because What Could Go Wrong with a Science Hive Mind?," The Federalist, May 11, 2022, https://thefederalist.com/2022/05/11/top-medical-licensure-board-creates-misinformation-policy-because-what-could-go-wrong-with-a-science-hive-mind/.
89. Augusto Del Noce, *The Crisis of Modernity*, trans. Carlo Lancelloti (Montreal: McGill-Queen's University Press, 2014), 232.
90. Agamben, *Where Are We Now?*, 49.
91. Del Noce, *Crisis of Modernity*, 89.
92. Sophocles's ancient Greek tragedy *Antigone* recounts the story of the daughter of Oedipus. The drama centers upon a decree from the King of Thebes that the rebels in the Theban civil war could not be given burial. The protagonist, Antigone, is torn between her civic duty to obey the king and her natural familial duty to bury her brother. "It is the dead, not the living, who make the longest demands," she laments. "We have only a little time to please the living. But all eternity to love the dead." She makes the anguishing but brave choice to defy the king's order and honor her brother with a burial. When brought before the king, Antigone admits she was aware that her action violated his decree but insists that she must follow divine law over human law. After condemning her to death, the king is eventually moved by her courage and decides to release her from prison. However, still unaware of the king's change of heart and just before she could be released, Antigone hangs herself to avoid death by stoning.
93. Eric Voegelin, "The Origins of Totalitarianism," *Review of Politics* 15, no. 1 (January 1953): 68–76, http://www.jstor.org/stable/1404747.
94. Del Noce, *Crisis of Modernity*, 153.
95. Ibid., 290.
96. Ibid., 90.
97. Ibid., 91.
98. Augusto Del Noce, *The Age of Secularization*, trans. Carlo Lancelloti (Montreal: McGill-Queen's University Press, 2017), 29.
99. Ibid., 85.
100. Ernst Nolte, *Three Faces of Fascism: Action Française, Italian Fascism, National Socialism* (New York: Mentor, 1969), 308–9.
101. This is a necessarily condensed sketch of my more extensive argument regarding these ideologies as ruptures with the past, presented in my article, "The Latent Fascism of Today's Anti-Fascists." Simone Weil Center for Political Philosophy, July 12, 2020, https://simoneweilcenter.org/publications/2021/2/14/the-latent-fascism-of-todays-anti-fascists.
102. Mattias Desmet, *The Psychology of Totalitarianism* (White River Junction: Chelsea Green, 2022).
103. For a summary of Desmet's theory of mass formation, as well as Rene Girard's theory of mimetic contagion and scapegoating, as applied to our collective social behavior during the pandemic, see my article: "Mass Formation, Mimetic Contagion, and Scapegoating," Human Flourishing (Substack), April 13, 2022, https://aaronkheriaty.substack.com/p/mass-formation-mimetic-contagion
104. Agamben, *Where Are We Now?*, 10–11.
105. Ibid., 58.

Chapter 2: Locked Down & Locked Out: A New Societal Paradigm

1. Kimiko de Freytas-Tamura, "Footage Reveals New Details in Tourist Melee at N.Y.C. Restaurant," *New York Times*, September 18, 2021, https://www.nytimes.com/2021/09/18/nyregion/carmines-vaccination-fight.html.

2. Joseph Goldstein and Matthew Sedacca, "Why Only 28 Percent of Young Black New Yorkers Are Vaccinated," *New York Times*, August 12, 2021, https://www.nytimes.com/2021/08/12/nyregion/covid-vaccine-black-young-new-yorkers.html.

3. Nick Corbishley, *Scanned: Why Vaccine Passports and Digital IDs Will Mean the End of Privacy and Personal Freedom* (White River Junction: Chelsea Green, 2022), 1.

4. Ibid., 94.

5. Michel Foucault, *Discipline & Punish: The Birth of the Prison*, trans. Alan Sheridan (New York: Vintage Books, 1995), 195–228.

6. Corbishley, *Scanned*, 21–22.

7. S. V. Subramanian and Akhil Kumar, "Increases in COVID-19 Are Unrelated to Levels of Vaccination across 68 Countries and 2947 Counties in the United States," *European Journal of Epidemiology* 36, no. 12 (2021): 1237–40, https://pubmed.ncbi.nlm.nih.gov/34591202/.

8. Sarah A. Buchan et al., "Effectiveness of COVID-19 Vaccines against Omicron or Delta Symptomatic Infection and Severe Outcomes," medRxiv (January 28, 2022), https://doi.org/10.1101/2021.12.30.21268565.

9. "WHO Warns against Blanket Boosters, as Vaccine Inequity Persists," United Nations, December 22, 2021, https://news.un.org/en/story/2021/12/1108622; Jemima McEvoy, "WHO Calls for Pause on Covid Booster Shots until 2022," *Forbes*, September 9, 2021, https://www.forbes.com/sites/jemimamcevoy/2021/09/08/who-calls-for-pause-on-covid-booster-shots-until-2022/?sh=426732257f9a.

10. UK Health Security Agency, *COVID-19 Vaccine Surveillance Report: Week 1* (London: UK Health Security Agency, 2022), https://assets.publishing.service.gov.uk/government/uploads/system/uploads/attachment_data/file/1045329/Vaccine_surveillance_report_week_1_2022.pdf; Frederik Plesner Lyngse et al., "SARS-CoV-2 Omicron VOC Transmission in Danish Households," medRxiv, December 27, 2021, https://doi.org/10.1101/2021.12.27.21268278; Christian Holm Hansen et al., "Vaccine Effectiveness against SARS-CoV-2 Infection with the Omicron or Delta Variants Following a Two-Dose or Booster BNT162b2 or mRNA-1273 Vaccination Series: A Danish Cohort Study," medRxiv, December 21, 2021, https://doi.org/10.1101/2021.12.20.21267966. For a summary of the key findings of these studies cf. Paul Alexander, "NEGATIVE EFFICACY: U.K. Health Agency First 'COVID-19 Vaccine Surveillance Report' of 2022, Collates Infection Rate Data for the Final Weeks of 2021 (Weeks 49–52); A DEVASTATING REPORT," Substack Alexander COVID News Evidence-Based Medicine (Substack), January 7, 2022, https://palexander.substack.com/p/uk-health-security-agency-first-covid?s=r&utm_campaign=post&utm_medium=web; cf. also, Alex Berenson, "Has Covid Vaccine Efficacy Turned Negative?," Unreported Truths (Substack), January 6, 2022, https://alexberenson.substack.com/p/has-covid-vaccine-efficacy-turned.

11. Heba N. Altarawneh et al., "Effects of Previous Infection and Vaccination on Symptomatic Omicron Infections," *New England Journal of Medicine* 387, no. 1 (2022): 21–34, https://www.nejm.org/doi/full/10.1056/NEJMoa2203965.

12. Apoorva Mandavilli, "The C.D.C. Isn't Publishing Large Portions of the Covid Data It Collects," *New York Times*, February 20, 2022, https://www.nytimes.com/2022/02/20/health/covid-cdc-data.html.

13. Oliver Barnes and John Burn-Murdoch, "Covid Infections Surge to Record-High for Over-70s in UK," *Financial Times*, March 16, 2022, https://www.ft.com/content/b4bf71b1-0b60-41fd-b445-ce13379a270c.

14. Helen McArdle, "Public Health Scotland Pulls Covid Case Rate Data over Claims It 'Demonstrates Conclusively' That Vaccines Are Not Working," *Herald of Scotland*, February 17, 2022, https://www.heraldscotland.com/news/19932323.public-health-scotland-pulls-covid-case-rate-data-claims-demonstrates-conclusively-vaccines-not-working/.

15. Allie Simon, "Calif. Colleges Demand COVID Booster Compliance: Shut Off WiFi, Threaten Punishments," The College Fix, April 1, 2022, https://www.thecollegefix.com/calif-colleges-demand-covid-booster-compliance-shut-off-wifi-threaten-punishments/.

16. "Fauci: 'We Should Not Get So Fixated on This Elusive Number of Herd Immunity,'" Grabien, March 15, 2021, https://grabien.com/story.php?id=328251.

17. Jaimy Lee, "Is Herd Immunity a Realistic Concept? Fauci Calls It 'Elusive' and 'Mystical,'" MarketWatch, May 7, 2021, https://www.marketwatch.com/story/is-herd-immunity-a-realistic-concept-fauci-calls-it-elusive-and-mystical-11620148465.

18. Ohio Department of Health, "What's in the Vaccine?," YouTube, April 16, 2021, https://www.youtube.com/watch?v=-Gg5ETxxspA.

19. Mandavilli, "The C.D.C. Isn't Publishing Large Portions."

20. Jesus Jiménez, "Washington State Allows for Free Marijuana with Covid-19 Vaccine," *New York Times*, June 7, 2021.

21. Aaron Kheriaty and Gerard V. Bradley, "University Vaccine Mandates Violate Medical Ethics," *Wall Street Journal*, June 14, 2021.

22. Ibid.

23. The entire panel is available for viewing at Senator Ron Johnson, "COVID-19: A SECOND Opinion," Rumble, January 24, 2022, https://rumble.com/vt62y6-covid-19-a-second-opinion.html. An edited version with my remarks is available at KanekoaTheGreat, "Dr. Aaron Kheriarty Full Highlights | Senator Ron Johnson COVID-19: A Second Opinion," Rumble, January 25, 2022, https://rumble.com/embed/vqmilm/?pub=4.

24. Johnson, "COVID-19"; KanekoaTheGreat, "Dr. Aaron Kheriarty."

25. Jonathan Isaac and Aaron Kheriaty, "COVID Mandates Prevent Americans from Getting Back in the Game," Fox News, January 10, 2022, https://www.foxnews.com/opinion/covid-coronavirus-vaccine-mandates-biden-nba-jonathan-isaac.

26. Kyle Harper, *The Fate of Rome: Climate, Disease, and the End of an Empire* (Princeton: Princeton University Press, 2019).

27. Michael Barbaro, Alexandra Leigh Young, Neena Pathak, Stella Tan, and Michael Simon Johnson, "The Coronavirus Goes Global," *The Daily*, February 27, 2020, https://www.nytimes.com/2020/02/27/podcasts/the-daily/coronavirus.html; Donald G. McNeil Jr., "To Take On the Coronavirus, Go Medieval on It," *New York Times*, February 28, 2020, https://www.nytimes.com/2020/02/28/sunday-review/coronavirus-quarantine.html.

28. Alex Gutentag, "The Great Covid Class War," The Bellows, December 16, 2020, https://www.thebellows.org/the-great-covid-class-war/.

29. Alex Berenson, "Fifteen Days," chapter 6 in *Pandemia: How Coronavirus Hysteria Took Over Our Government, Rights, and Lives* (Washington, D.C.: Regnery Publishing, 2021).

30. Aaron Kheriaty, "The Impossible Ethics of Pandemic Triage," *New Atlantis*, April 3, 2020, https://www.thenewatlantis.com/publications/the-impossible-ethics-of-pandemic-triage.

31. Mariana Mazzucato, "Avoiding a Climate Lockdown," Project Syndicate, September 22, 2020, https://www.project-syndicate.org/commentary/radical-green-overhaul-to-avoid-climate-lockdown-by-mariana-mazzucato-2020-09.

32. Gutentag, "Great Covid Class War."

33. Jonas Herby, Lars Jonung, and Steve H. Hanke, "A Literature Review and Meta-Analysis of the Effects of Lockdowns on COVID-19 Mortality," *Studies in Applied Economics* no. 200 (January 2022): 2.

34. Ibid.

35. World Health Organization, *Report of the WHO-China Joint Mission on Coronavirus Disease 2019 (COVID-19)* (Geneva: World Health Organization, 2020), https://www.who.int/publications/i/item/report-of-the-who-china-joint-mission-on-coronavirus-disease-2019-(covid-19), 19.

36. Jan Jekeliek, "Jeffrey Tucker: How the US Adopted CCP-Inspired COVID-19 Control Policies, a Timeline," *Epoch Times*, May 7, 2022, https://www.theepochtimes.com/jeffrey-tucker-how-the-us-adopted-ccp-inspired-covid-19-control-policies-a-timeline_4440770.html.

37. Jeffrey A. Tucker, "The China Model Unravels in Shanghai," Brownstone Institute, April 11, 2022, https://brownstone.org/articles/the-china-model-unravels-in-shanghai/.

38. "About WHO," World Health Organization, 2022, https://www.who.int/about/.

39. Oona Hathaway and Alasdair Phillips-Robins, " COVID-19 and International Law Series: Reforming the World Health Organization," Just Security, December 11, 2020, https://www.justsecurity.org/73793/covid-19-and-international-law-series-reforming-the-world-health-organization/

40. Associated Press, "WHO Chief Praises China's Virus Fight, Urges More from World," Yahoo! News, February 15, 2020, https://nz.news.yahoo.com/chief-praises-chinas-virus-fight-145551598.html; "Statement on the Second Meeting of the International Health Regulations (2005) Emergency Committee regarding the Outbreak of Novel Coronavirus (2019-nCoV)," World Health Organization, January 30, 2020, https://www.who.int/news/item/30-01-2020-statement-on-the-second-meeting-of-the-international-health-regulations-(2005)-emergency-committee-regarding-the-outbreak-of-novel-coronavirus-(2019-ncov).

41. Tedros Adhanom Ghebreyesus (@DrTedros), "In many ways, #China is actually setting a new standard . . . ," Twitter, January 30, 2020, 4:40 p.m., https://twitter.com/DrTedros/status/1222982869871669251.

42. Freddie Sayers, "Neil Ferguson Interview: China Changed What Was Possible," UnHerd, December 26, 2020, https://unherd.com/thepost/neil-ferguson-interview-china-changed-what-was-possible/.

43. Andrew Scheuber, "Chinese President Sees UK-China Academic Partnerships at Imperial," Imperial College London, October 21, 2015, https://www.imperial.ac.uk/news/168497/chinese-president-sees-ukchina-academic-partners-hips/.

44. Tucker, "The China Model Unravels."

45. "Shanghai Lockdown Risks Becoming Biggest Crisis of Xi's Tenure," Bloomberg, April 7, 2022, https://www.bloomberg.com/news/articles/2022-04-07/shanghai-lockdown-risks-becoming-biggest-crisis-of-xi-s-tenure.

46. Joe Wang, "Desperation and Despotism in Shanghai," Brownstone Institute, May 7, 2022, https://brownstone.org/articles/desperation-and-despotism-in-shanghai/.

47. Ibid.

48. "Covid Zero Defended in China as Shanghai Cases Top 21,000," Bloomberg, April 7, 2022, https://www.bloomberg.com/news/articles/2022-04-08/china-s-covid-zero-policy-defended-as-shanghai-frustration-grows#xj4y7vzkg.

49. CNBC Television, "Shanghai Patient Mistaken for Dead Sparks 'Lockdown' Horror," YouTube, May 2, 2022, https://youtu.be/lMGjcr3aAak.

50. Aaron Kheriaty, MD (@akheriaty), "Biomedical security state, Chinese edition. Shanghai lockdowns . . . ," Twitter, April 24, 2022, 11:59 a.m., https://twitter.com/akheriaty/status/1518243297101111298; Aaron Kheriaty, MD (@akheriaty), "Biomedical security state, Chinese edition . . . ," Twitter, April 17, 2022, 3:35 p.m., https://twitter.com/akheriaty/status/1515760838115618818.

51. Corbishley, *Scanned*, 57–58.

52. Alyssa Rosenburg, "The Baby Formula Shortage Is an Outrage. A Sane Country Would Fix It," *Washington Post*, May 10, 2022, https://www.washingtonpost.com/opinions/2022/05/10/abbott-baby-formula-shortage-needs-solutions/.

53. Aaron Kheriaty, "The Other Pandemic: The Lockdown Mental Health Crisis," Public Discourse, October 4, 2020, https://www.thepublicdiscourse.com/2020/10/71969/.

54. Ibid.

55. Mark É. Czeisler et al., "Mental Health, Substance Use, and Suicidal Ideation during the COVID-19 Pandemic—United States, June 24–30, 2020," *Morbidity and Mortality Weekly Report*, 69, no. 32 (2020): 1049–57, https://www.cdc.gov/mmwr/volumes/69/wr/mm6932a1.htm?s_cid=mm6932a1_w; Kheriaty, "The Other Pandemic."

56. Kheriaty, "The Other Pandemic."

57. "Multiple Causes of Death 1999–2020," CDC Wonder, December 2021, https://wonder.cdc.gov/wonder/help/mcd.html; Aaron Kheriaty, MD (@akheriaty), "The other pandemic . . . ," Twitter, March 24, 2022, 8:11 p.m., https://twitter.com/akheriaty/status/1507132969487462422.

58. Aaron M. White et al., "Alcohol-Related Deaths during the COVID-19 Pandemic," *Journal of the American Medical Association* 327, no. 17 (2022): 1704–6, https://jamanetwork.com/journals/jama/fullarticle/2790491.

59. Lucy Craft, "Suicide Claimed More Japanese Lives in October Than 10 Months of COVID," CBS News, November 13, 2020, https://www.cbsnews.com/news/japan-suicide-coronavirus-more-japanese-suicides-in-october-than-total-covid-deaths/.

60. William Wan, "Pandemic Isolation Has Killed Thousands of Alzheimer's Patients while Families Watch from Afar," *Washington Post*, September 16, 2020, https://www.washingtonpost.com/health/2020/09/16/coronavirus-dementia-alzheimers-deaths/.

61. Ann Case and Angus Deaton, *Deaths of Despair and the Future of Capitalism* (Princeton: Princeton University Press, 2021); cf. also Aaron Kheriaty, "Dying of Despair," *First Things* no. 275 (August/September 2017), https://www.firstthings.com/article/2017/08/dying-of-despair.

62. Houston Community College, "COVID-19 PSA—Alone Together," YouTube, May 24, 2020, https://www.youtube.com/watch?v=JjVUzY6lSRA.

63. Hannah Arendt, *The Origins of Totalitarianism* (New York: Harcourt Brace Jovanovich, 1973), 478.

64. White et al., "Alcohol-Related Deaths."

65. Luke Money, Matt Stiles, and Colleen Shalby, "California's Secret Weapon in COVID-19 Success: We Are Not Skeptical about the Vaccine," *Los Angeles Times*, May 1, 2021, https://www.latimes.com/california/story/2021-05-01/minimal-vaccine-hesitancy-fuels-californias-covid-recovery; Collen Shalby and Hayley Smith, "California's Huge COVID-19 Vaccine Expansion Relies on Trust. Will Cheaters Stay Away?," *Los Angeles Times*, March 16, 2021, https://www.latimes.com/california/story/2021-03-16/californias-covid-19-vaccine-expansion-relies-on-honor-system-you-have-to-try-to-trust.

66. Kristie E. N. Clarke et al., "Seroprevalence of Infection-Induced SARS-CoV-2 Antibodies—United States, September 2021–February 2022," *Morbidity and Mortality Weekly Report*, 71, no. 17 (2022): 606–8, https://www.cdc.gov/mmwr/volumes/71/wr/mm7117e3.htm.

67. Sivan Gazit et al., "SARS-CoV-2 Naturally Acquired Immunity vs. Vaccine-Induced Immunity, Reinfections versus Breakthrough Infections: A Retrospective Cohort Study," *Clinical Infectious Diseases* (2022), https://www.ncbi.nlm.nih.gov/pmc/articles/PMC9047157/pdf/ciac262.pdf.

68. Shai Efrati et al., "Safety and Humoral Responses to BNT162b2 mRNA Vaccination of SARS-CoV-2 Previously Infected and Naive Populations," *Scientific Reports* 11, 16543 (2021), https://doi.org/10.1038/s41598-021-96129-6; Rachel K. Raw et al., "Previous COVID-19 Infection but Not Long-COVID Is Associated with Increased Adverse Events Following BNT162b2/Pfizer Vaccination," *Journal of Infection*, 83, no. 3 (September 2021): 381–412, https://doi.org/10.1101/2021.04.15.21252192; Noam Barda et al., "Safety of the BNT162b2 mRNA Covid-19 Vaccine in a Nationwide Setting," *New England Journal of Medicine* 385 no. 12 (2021): 1078–90, https://www.nejm.org/doi/pdf/10.1056/NEJMoa2110475?articleTools=true; Cristina Menni et al., "Vaccine Side-Effects and SARS-CoV-2 Infection after Vaccination in Users of the COVID Symptom Study App in the UK: A Prospective Observational Study," *Lancet Infectious Diseases* 21, no. 7 (2021): 939–49, https://doi.org/10.1016/S1473-3099(21)00224-3.

69. Andrew Bostom et. al, "How College COVID Vaccine Mandates Put Students in Danger," The Federalist, July 5, 2021, https://thefederalist.com/2021/07/05/how-college-covid-vaccine-mandates-put-students-in-danger/.

70. Ibid.

71. Aaron Kheriaty, "The Physician's Vocation," Mercatornet, September 14, 2018, https://mercatornet.com/the-physicians-vocation/23584/.

72. After my dismissal, support came from places I had not expected. You learn who your friends are when you undergo trials. A professor of English at UCLA, whom I had not met prior to my dismissal, was among the strangers who reached out to encourage me. He wrote a letter to the UCI chancellor explaining, "Although I have neither worked nor met with Dr. Kheriaty, I have profited tremendously not only from his academic work on bioethics but also from his current public-facing writings on informed consent and bio-surveillance (and will be teaching one of his essays in the Fall)." I was surprised and

edified that he said, "I can hardly overstate the fact that Dr. Kheriaty has impacted my own pedagogy in ways that few other teachers have."

This colleague went on to say, "Dr. Kheriaty is the rare teacher who dared to exhibit the courage of informed conviction outside the classroom. Despite his firing, he continues to represent and inspire many others at our University who found themselves to be passive objects of communication rather than active subjects in communication on matters related to Covid protocols." He concluded, "The summary firing of Dr. Kheriaty, a full professor in the School of Medicine, has shaken me to the very core: not just me but also those who care deeply for our University's commitment to academic freedom and the spirit of inquiry."

This professor was not the only one willing to speak publicly. A former vice chancellor and son of the founding chancellor of UCI also wrote a letter on my behalf. He cited historical examples in which the University of California, Irvine, had compromised on its commitments by unjustly firing faculty. He mentioned the loyalty oath of the 1950s "that attacked academic freedom and led to the termination of faculty like Dr. David Saxson," who was reinstated and went on to become provost at UCLA and subsequently president of the University of California. He also mentioned the edifying example of a previous chancellor who stood by Professor Sherwood Rowland amidst intense pressure from corporate interests and other scientists to remove him. That decision was later vindicated when Professor Rowland won the Nobel Prize in chemistry. Clearly, good ideas are not always embraced by the scientific community immediately when they are introduced.

However far the institutional corruption at our universities has progressed, I am grateful that there are still many good people like these in academia. Our students deserve no less. Besides missing the students and residents, I also miss working with colleagues like these who remain dedicated to the highest ideals of the university, whatever the challenges. But I also worry that the corruption in our universities has reached a terminal stage. Higher education is in serious crisis, as is now widely acknowledged. In the aftermath, new educational institutions will need to be built upon these ruins.

73. *Jacobson v. Massachusetts*, 197 U.S. 11 (1905), https://supreme.justia.com/cases/federal/us/197/11/.
74. "Smallpox," Centers for Disease Control and Prevention, https://www.cdc.gov/smallpox/clinicians/clinical-disease.html.
75. *Buck v. Bell*, 274 U.S. 200 (1927), https://supreme.justia.com/cases/federal/us/274/200/.
76. Mattias Desmet, *The Psychology of Totalitarianism* (White River Junction: Chelsea Green, 2022), 81.
77. Clarke et al., "Seroprevalence of Infection-Induced SARS-CoV-2 Antibodies."
78. John P. A. Ioannidis, Cathrine Axfors, and Despina G. Contopoulos-Ioannidis, "Population-Level COVID-19 Mortality Risk for Non-Elderly Individuals Overall and for Non-Elderly Individuals without Underlying Diseases in Pandemic Epicenters, *Environmental Research* 188, no. 109890 (2020), https://doi.org/10.1016/j.envres.2020.109890; John P. A. Ioannidis, "Infection Fatality Rate of COVID-19 Inferred from Seroprevalence Data," *Bulletin World Health Organization* 99, no. 1 (2021): 19–33, http://dx.doi.org/10.2471/BLT.20.265892.
79. Ioannidis, Axfors, and Contopoulos-Ioannidis, "Population-Level COVID-19 Mortality Risk"; Ioannidis, "Infection Fatality Rate of COVID-19."
80. Sarah Tanveer et al, "Transparency of COVID-19 Vaccine Trials: Decisions without Data," *BMJ Evidence-Based Medicine*, August 9, 2021, https://ebm.bmj.com/content/early/2021/08/08/bmjebm-2021-111735.
81. "Public Health and Medical Professionals for Transparency," 2022, https://phmpt.org/.
82. Hugh Black et al., "Allocation of Scarce Critical Resources under Crisis Standards of Care," UC Bioethics Working Group, June 17, 2020, https://www.ucop.edu/uc-health/reports-resources/uc-critical-care-bioethics-working-group-report-rev-6-17-20.pdf.
83. *PHMPT v. FDA*, No. 21-1058 (N.D. Tex. 2022).
84. "5.3.6 CUMULATIVE ANALYSIS OF POST-AUTHORIZATION ADVERSE EVENT REPORTS OF PF-07302048 (BNT162B2) RECEIVED THROUGH 28-FEB-2021," PHMPT, February 28, 2021, https://phmpt.org/wp-content/uploads/2021/11/5.3.6-postmarketing-experience.pdf
85. Ibid.

86. Rebecca Strong, "Putting Big Bad Pharma Back on Trial in the COVID-19 Era," Medium, February 16, 2021, https://medium.com/@bexstrong/big-pharma-corruption-and-lawsuits-amidst-covid-vaccine-c734a494b776.

87. Chris Pandolfo, "The Federal Government Paid Hundreds of Media Companies to Advertise the COVID-19 Vaccines while Those Same Outlets Provided Positive Coverage of the Vaccines," Blaze Media, March 3, 2022, https://www.theblaze.com/news/review-the-federal-government-paid-media-companies-to-advertise-for-the-vaccines.

88. Strong, "Putting Big Bad Pharma Back on Trial."

89. Ibid.

90. Charles Piller, "Is FDA's Revolving Door Open Too Wide?," *Science* 361, no. 6397 (July 2018): 21, https://www.science.org/doi/full/10.1126/science.361.6397.21.

91. Jeffrey Bien and Vinay Prasad, "Future Jobs of FDA's Haematology-Oncology Reviewers," *British Medical Journal* 354, no. i5055 (2016), https://doi.org/10.1136/bmj.i5055.

92. Maryanne Demasi, "From FDA to MHRA: Are Drug Regulators for Hire?" *British Medical Journal* 377, no. o1538 (2022), https://www.bmj.com/content/bmj/377/bmj.o1538.full.pdf.

93. Joel Achenbach, "NIH Halts $100 Million Study of Moderate Drinking That Is Funded by Alcohol Industry," *Washington Post*, May 18, 2018, https://www.washingtonpost.com/news/to-your-health/wp/2018/05/17/nih-halts-controversial-study-of-moderate-drinking/.

94. Alexander Tin, "Moderna Offers NIH Co-Ownership of COVID Vaccine Patent amid Dispute with Government," CBS News, November 15, 2021, https://www.cbsnews.com/news/moderna-covid-vaccine-patent-dispute-national-institutes-health/.

95. "NIH Officials Profiting from COVID-19 Vaccine," Informed Consent Action Network, 2021, https://www.icandecide.org/nih-officials-profiting-from-covid-19-vaccine/.

96. Adam Andrzejewski, "Substack Investigation: Fauci's Royalties and the $350 Million Royalty Payment Stream HIDDEN by NIH," Open the Books, May 16, 2022, https://www.openthebooks.com/substack-investigation-faucis-royalties-and-the-350-million-royalty-payment-stream-hidden-by-nih/.

97. Judith Garber, "CDC 'Disclaimers' Hide Financial Conflicts of Interest," Lown Institute, November 6, 2019, https://lowninstitute.org/cdc-disclaimers-hide-financial-conflicts-of-interest/; see also "Citizen Petition to CDC," U.S. Right to Know, September 5, 2019, https://usrtk.org/wp-content/uploads/2019/11/Petition-to-CDC-re-Disclaimers.pdf.

98. Caroline Chen, "FDA Repays Industry by Rushing Risky Drugs to Market," ProPublica, June 26, 2018, https://www.propublica.org/article/fda-repays-industry-by-rushing-risky-drugs-to-market.

99. Strong, "Putting Big Bad Pharma Back."

100. Søren Ventegodt, "Why the Corruption of the World Health Organization (WHO) Is the Biggest Threat to the World's Public Health of Our Time," Journal of Integrative Medicine & Therapy 2, no. 1 (2015): 5; K. M. Gopakumar, "WHO: Do Financial Contributions from 'Pharma' Violate WHO Guidelines," Third World Network, December 8, 2015, https://archive.globalpolicy.org/home/270-general/52830-who-do-financial-contributions-from-pharma-violate-who-guidelines.html; Deidre McPhillips, "Gates Foundation Donations to WHO Nearly Match Those from U.S. Government," *U.S. News and World Report*, May 29, 2020, https://www.usnews.com/news/articles/2020-05-29/gates-foundation-donations-to-who-nearly-match-those-from-us-government; cf. also Strong, "Putting Big Bad Pharma Back."

101. Catherine Cheney, "'Big Concerns' over Gates Foundation's Potential to Become Largest WHO Donor," Devex, June 5, 2020, https://www.devex.com/news/big-concerns-over-gates-foundation-s-potential-to-become-largest-who-donor-97377.

102. "Our Partners," CDC Foundation, 2022, https://www.cdcfoundation.org/partner-list/corporations.

103. Paul Thacker, "Covid-19: Researcher Blows the Whistle on Data Integrity Issues in Pfizer's Vaccine Trial," *British Medical Journal* 375, no. n2635 (2021), https://pubmed.ncbi.nlm.nih.gov/34728500/.

104. Strong, "Putting Big Bad Pharma Back."

105. Fernando Polack et al., "Safety and Efficacy of the BNT162b2 mRNA Covid-19 Vaccine," *New England Journal of Medicine* 383, no. 27 (December 2020): 2603–15, https://www.ncbi.nlm.nih.gov/pmc/articles/PMC7745181/.
106. Strong, "Putting Big Bad Pharma Back."
107. David Healy, "Disappeared in Argentina," Dr. David Healy, March 1, 2022, https://davidhealy.org/disappeared-in-argentina/.
108. Josh Guetzkow, "Is Subject #12312982 the Key to Proving Pfizer Vaccine Trial Fraud?: The Story of Augusto Roux," Jackanapes Junction (Substack), May 22, 2022, https://jackanapes.substack.com/p/is-subject-12312982-the-key-to-proving?s=r.
109. Ibid.
110. Healy, "Disappeared in Argentina."
111. Ibid.

Chapter 3: Locked In: The Coming Technocratic Dystopia

1. Cited in Nick Corbishley, *Scanned: Why Vaccine Passports, Mandates, and Digital IDs Will Mean the End of Privacy and Personal Freedom* (Hartford, Vermont: Chelsea Green, 2022), 72.
2. George Orwell, *Nineteen Eighty-Four* (London: Secker and Warburg, 1949), 155.
3. Caylan Ford, "Like COVID-19, Digital Passports Could Be with Us Forever," The Hub, November 19, 2021, https://thehub.ca/2021-11-19/caylan-ford-like-covid-digital-passports-could-be-with-us-forever/.
4. Allison Gardner, "Contact-Tracing Apps: There's No Evidence They're Helping Stop COVID-19," The Conversation, October 21, 2020, https://theconversation.com/contact-tracing-apps-theres-no-evidence-theyre-helping-stop-covid-19-148397
5. Luke Kemp, "The 'Stomp Reflex': When Governments Abuse Emergency Powers," BBC, April 28, 2021, https://www.bbc.com/future/article/20210427-the-stomp-reflex-when-governments-abuse-emergency-powers.
6. Madhumita Murgia, "England's NHS Plans to Share Patient Records with Third Parties," *Financial Times*, May 26, 2021, https://www.ft.com/content/9fee812f-6975-49ce-915c-aeb25d3dd748.
7. Madhumita Murgia and Max Harlow, "NHS Shares English Hospital Data with Dozens of Companies," *Financial Times*, July 26, 2021, https://www.ft.com/content/6f9f6f1f-e2d1-4646-b5ec-7d704e45149e.
8. Rob Davies, "NHS App Storing Facial Verification Data via Contract with Firm Linked to Tory Donors," *The Guardian*, September 15, 2021, https://www.theguardian.com/society/2021/sep/15/nhs-app-storing-facial-verification-data-via-contract-with-firm-linked-to-tory-donors.
9. George Orwell, "Politics and the English Language," *Horizon* no. 76 (April 1946).
10. George Orwell, *Nineteen Eighty-Four* (London: Secker and Warburg, 1949), 29–30.
11. Ibid., 126.
12. Ibid., 18–19.
13. Giorgio Agamben, *Where Are We Now: The Pandemic as Politics* (London: Rowman & Littlefield, 2021), 75.
14. Ibid, 77.
15. Klaus Schwab and Thierry Malleret, *COVID-19: The Great Reset* (Geneva: World Economic Forum, 2020).
16. Ibid., 12.
17. Ibid., 142.
18. Ibid., 93.
19. C. S. Lewis, *The Abolition of Man* (New York: HarperCollins, 2015).
20. Corbishley, *Scanned*, 52–53.
21. Peter S. Goodman, *Davos Man: How the Billionaires Devoured the World* (New York: Custom House, 2022).
22. Ibid.
23. Alex Gutentag, "Revolt of the Essential Workers," Tablet, October 25, 2021, https://www.tabletmag.com/sections/news/articles/revolt-essential-workers.

24. Carol Roth, "Lockdowns Were a Gift to Big Business Designed to Kill Small Biz," *New York Post*, July 5, 2021, https://nypost.com/2021/07/05/lockdowns-were-a-gift-to-big-biz-designed-to-kill-small-biz/.

25. Gutentag, "Revolt of the Essential Workers."

26. Alex Gutentag, "The Great Covid Class War," The Bellows, December 16, 2020, https://www.thebellows.org/the-great-covid-class-war/.

27. Goodman, *Davos Man*.

28. Andrew Stuttaford, "The Great Reset: If Only It Were Just a Conspiracy," *National Review*, November 27, 2020, https://www.nationalreview.com/2020/11/the-great-reset-if-only-it-were-just-a-conspiracy/.

29. Iain Davis, "What Is the 'Global Public-Private Partnership'?" OffGuardian, October 20, 2021, https://off-guardian.org/2021/10/20/what-is-the-global-public-private-partnership/.

30. Joan Dzenowagis and Gael Kernen, *Connecting for Health: Global Vision, Local Insight; Report for the World Summit on the Information Society* (Switzerland: World Health Organization, 2005), available via the WayBack Machine at https://web.archive.org/web/20210403084237/https://apps.who.int/iris/bitstream/handle/10665/43385/9241593903_eng.pdf?sequence=1&isAllowed=y.

31. Schwab and Malleret, *COVID-19*.

32. Ibid., 92.

33. Michael Rectenwald, "What Is the Great Reset?," Michael Rectenwald , November 7, 2021, https://www.michaelrectenwald.com/great-reset-essays-interviews/what-is-the-great-reset.

34. Giorgio Agamben, "Communist Capitalism," trans. Richard Braude, Ill Will, December 15, 2020, https://illwill.com/communist-capitalism.

35. Ibid.

36. Cited in Schwab and Malleret, *COVID-19*.

37. "World Health Assembly Agrees to Launch Process to Develop Historic Global Accord on Pandemic Prevention, Preparedness and Response," World Health Organization, December 1, 2021, https://www.who.int/news/item/01-12-2021-world-health-assembly-agrees-to-launch-process-to-develop-historic-global-accord-on-pandemic-prevention-preparedness-and-response. The working group report can be found at World Health Organization, *Report of the Member States Working Group on Strengthening WHO Preparedness and Response to Health Emergencies to the Special Session of the World Health Assembly* (Geneva: World Health Organization, 2021), https://apps.who.int/gb/ebwha/pdf_files/WHASSA2/SSA2_3-en.pdf.

38. Keean Bexte, "#StopTheTreaty: WHO Allows Brief Feedback on Global Pandemic Treaty," The Counter Signal, April 12, 20221, https://thecountersignal.com/who-allows-brief-feed-back-on-global-pandemic-treaty/.

39. "Strengthening WHO Preparedness for and Response to Health Emergencies," World Health Organization, April 12, 2022, https://apps.who.int/gb/ebwha/pdf_files/WHA75/A75_18-en.pdf.

40. Ibid., 8.

41. "The WHO Pandemic Treaty and Our Health Care Sovereignty," Leslyn Lewis, https://leslynlewis.ca/blog/the-who-pandemic-treaty-and-our-health-care-sovereignty/.

42. Albert Hold, "Checking Covid 19 Certificates: World Health Organization Selects T-Systems as Industry Partner," Telekom, February 23, 2022, https://www.telekom.com/en/media/media-information/archive/covid-19-who-commissions-t-systems-648634.

43. Connie Chen and Emily Hochberg, "CLEAR Is One of the Best Ways to Skip Airport Lines, and It's Easier to Sign Up Than TSA Precheck," Business Insider, October 6, 2021, https://www.insider.com/guides/travel/clear-airport-security-review-how-it-works.

44. ID2020, "Immunization: An Entry Point for Digital Identity," Medium, March 28, 2018, https://medium.com/id2020/immunization-an-entry-point-for-digital-identity-ea37d9c3b77e.

45. Seth Berkley, "Immunization Needs a Technology Boost," *Nature* 551, no. 273 (2017), https://doi.org/10.1038/d41586-017-05923-8.

46. ID2020, "Immunization."

47. Corbishley, *Scanned*, 95.

48. John Thornhill, "India's All-Encompassing ID System Holds Warnings for the Rest of the World," *Financial Times*, November 11, 2021, https://www.ft.com/content/337f6d6e-7301-4ef4-a26d-a4e62f602947.

49. Varshi Rani, "Another City Is Using Crime Control as an Excuse for Facial Recognition Surveillance," *Vice,* November 27, 2020, https://www.vice.com/en/article/n7ve4q/varanasi-india-using-facial-recognition-surveillance-technology.

50. Liza Lin and Newley Purnell, "A World with a Billion Cameras Watching You Is Just around the Corner," *Wall Street Journal*, December 6, 2019, https://www.wsj.com/articles/a-billion-surveillance-cameras-forecast-to-be-watching-within-two-years-11575565402; cf. Corbishley, *Scanned*, 119–20.

51. Corbishley, *Scanned*, 105.

52. Tobias Adrian and Tommaso Mancini-Griffoli, "A New Era of Digital Money," International Monetary Fund, June 2021, https://www.imf.org/external/pubs/ft/fandd/2021/06/online/digital-money-new-era-adrian-mancini-griffoli.htm.

53. Alex Gutentag, "The Great Reset Is Real," Compact, March 22, 2022, https://compactmag.com/article/the-great-reset-is-real.

54. Shoshana Zuboff, *The Age of Surveillance Capitalism: The Fight for a Human Future at the New Frontier of Power* (New York: PublicAffairs, 2019).

55. Patrick Deneen, "The Unholy Marriage of Marx and Ayn Rand," Compact, April 22, 2022, https://compactmag.com/article/the-unholy-marriage-of-marx-and-ayn-rand.

56. Ibid.

57. "China Releases e-Yuan Cryptocurrency and Investors Are Going All-In," Yahoo! Finance, May 20, 2020, https://finance.yahoo.com/news/china-releases-e-yuan-cryptocurrency-180000183.html.

58. David Gura, "The U.S. Is Considering a Radical Rethinking of the Dollar for Today's Digital World" NPR, February 6, 2022, https://www.npr.org/2022/02/06/1072406109/digital-dollar-federal-reserve-apple-pay-venmo-cbdc.

59. Gutentag, "The Great Reset Is Real."

60. Douglas Farrow, "Whether There is a Moral Obligation to Disobey the Coercive Mandates," Theopolis Institute, January 27, 2022, https://theopolisinstitute.com/conversations/whether-there-is-a-moral-obligation-to-disobey-the-coercive-mandates/.

61. Balzé Halzé, "Yuval Noah Harari: 'Covid Is Critical . . . to Legitimize Total Biometric Surveillance," YouTube, May 21, 2022, https://www.youtube.com/watch?v=BoRMdsEnwBM&t=130s.

62. Ibid.

63. Ibid.

64. Ibid.

65. Ibid.

66. "Yuval Noah Harari: Covid-19 May Bring New Surveillance Era," BBC News, April 28, 2020, https://www.bbc.com/news/av/technology-52441339.

67. World Economic Forum, "Will the Future Be Human?—Yuval Noah Harari," YouTube, January 25, 2018, https://www.youtube.com/watch?v=hL9uk4hKyg4.

68. "Transhumanism—Klaus Schwab and Dr. Yuval Noah Harari Explain the Great Reset / Transhumanism Agenda," Rumble, February 8, 2022, https://rumble.com/vufrgx-tranhumanism-klaus-schwab-and-dr.-yuval-noah-harari-explain-the-great-reset.html.

69. World Economic Forum, "Will the Future Be Human?"

70. Athens Democracy Forum, "Dialogue: The Geopolitics of Technology," YouTube, October 6, 2021, https://youtu.be/KlFMEeOer3E.

71. Red Voice Media, "Harari: Useless People—Religious Ideas from Silicon Valley Will Take Over the World," Rumble, April 8, 2022, https://rumble.com/v1oaxoy-harari-useless-peoplereligious-ideas-from-silicon-valley-will-take-over-the.html.

72. Ibid.

73. Yuval Noah Harari, "Will the Future Be Human?—Yuval Noah Harari at the WEF Annual Meeting 2018," YouTube, January 31, 2018, https://www.youtube.com/watch?v=npfShBTNp3Q.

74. C. S. Lewis, *That Hideous Strength* (New York: HarperCollins, 1945), 169–70.

75. Ibid.

76. Christine Stabell Benn et al., "Randomised Clinical Trials of COVID-19 Vaccines: Do Adenovirus-Vector Vaccines Have Beneficial Non-Specific Effects?," preprints with *The Lancet*, April 5, 2022, http://dx.doi.org/10.2139/ssrn.4072489.

77. T. J. Britt et al., *Group Life COVID-19 Mortality Survey Report* (Schaumburg, Illinois: SOA Research Institute, 2022), https://www.soa.org/globalassets/assets/files/resources/research-report/2022/group-life-covid-19-mortality.pdf.

78. Markus Aldén et al., "Intracellular Reverse Transcription of Pfizer BioNTech COVID-19 mRNA Vaccine BNT162b2 In Vitro in Human Liver Cell Line," *Current Issues in Molecular Biology* 44, no. 3 (2022): 1115–26, https://www.mdpi.com/1467-3045/44/3/73/htm#B39-cimb-44-00073.

79. "Technology Futurist, Geopolitics Expert, Entrepreneur, Sci-Fi Novelist, Keynote Speaker," Jamie Metzl, https://jamiemetzl.com/.

80. Jamie Metzl, "Miraculous mRNA Vaccines Are Only the Beginning," *Newsweek*, February 12, 2021, https://www.newsweek.com/miraculous-mrna-vaccines-are-only-beginning-opinion-1567683.

81. Leon R. Kass, *Life, Liberty, and the Defense of Dignity: The Challenge for Bioethics* (New York: Encounter Books, 2004), 4.

82. Metzl, "Miraculous mRNA Vaccines."

83. Cf. Eugene McCarraher, *The Enchantments of Mammon: How Capitalism Became the Religion of Modernity* (Cambridge, Massachussetts: Harvard Belknap Press, 2019), 487.

84. Stefano Zamagni, "A Talk for the Simone Weil Center on Pandemic and Technocracy," Simone Weil Center, October 28, 2021, https://simoneweilcenter.org/publications/2021/10/28/a-talk-for-the-simone-weil-center-on-pandemic-and-technocracy. My panel discussion with Zamagni and others is available at SWC, "Simone Weil Center: Technocracy and the Pandemic, featuring Gov. Jerry Brown, Dr. Jay Battarcharya," YouTube, October 6, 2021, https://www.youtube.com/watch?v=AQzcfyMtPRU&t=215s.

85. Zamagni, "A Talk for the Simone Weil Center."

86. Ibid.

87. Ibid.

88. Augusto Del Noce, *The Crisis of Modernity*, trans. Carlo Lancellotti (Montreal: McGill-Queen's University Press, 2014), 24.

89. Ibid.

90. Gutentag, "The Great Covid Class War."

91. Jonathan Lange, "We Didn't Love Freedom Enough," *Kemmerer Gazette*, July 9, 2020, https://kemmerergazette.com/article/we-didnt-love-freedom-enough.

Chapter 4: Reclaiming Freedom: Human Flourishing in a More Rooted Future

1. Aaron Kheriaty, "Biosecurity Surveillance Regime: The Resistance, Part 1," Human Flourishing (Substack), December 19, 2021, https://aaronkheriaty.substack.com/p/biosecurity-surveillance-regime-the.

2. Corbishley, *Scanned*, 83.

3. Kheriaty, "Biosecurity Surveillance Regime"; Bruno Maçães, "Only Surveillance Can Save Us from Coronavirus," *Foreign Policy*, April 10, 2020, https://foreignpolicy.com/2020/04/10/coronavirus-pandemic-surveillance-privacy-big-data/.

4. Rowan (@canmericanized), "Canada Proud—Pro freedom anti mandate demonstrators pause in front of Toronto's Eaton Centre to sing the national anthem," Twitter, February 19, 2022, 4:13 p.m., https://twitter.com/canmericanized/status/1495144540293980164.

5. Ian Miles Cheong (@stillgray), "Remember this image. Remember what Trudeau did to Canada," Twitter, February 18, 2022, 6:52 p.m., https://twitter.com/stillgray/status/1494822254835765248.

6. Ezra Levant (@ezralevant), "1. I just spoke with Alexa Lavoie, our brave reporter who was just assaulted by Trudeau's police . . . ," Twitter, February 19, 2022, 10:46 a.m., https://twitter.com/ezralevant/status/1495062352735186944.

7. Darrell Bricker, "Nearly Half (46%) of Canadians Say They 'May Not Agree with Everything' Trucker Convoy Says or Does, But . . . ," Ipsos, February 11, 2022, https://

www.ipsos.com/en-ca/news-polls/nearly-half-say-they-may-not-agree-with-trucker-convoy.

8. Steve Scherer, "Pandemic Fatigue a Challenge for Canada's Trudeau amid Protests," *U.S. News and World Report*, February 17, 2022, https://www.usnews.com/news/world/articles/2022-02-17/analysis-pandemic-fatigue-a-challenge-for-canadas-trudeau-amid-protests.

9. Nate Hochman, "What the Ottawa Trucker Convoy Achieved," *National Review*, February 26, 2022, https://www.nationalreview.com/2022/02/what-the-ottawa-trucker-convoy-achieved/#slide-1.

10. James Roguski, "We Won," James Roguski (Substack), May 28, 2022, https://jamesroguski.substack.com/p/we-won.

11. Martin Heidegger, *Being and Time*, trans. Joan Stambaugh and Dennis Schmidt (Albany: State University of New York Press, 2010), 137.

12. Michel de Montaigne, *Selected Essays*, trans. James Atkinson and David Sices (Indianapolis: Hackett, 2012), 17.

13. In 2015 I ruptured a disk, which was followed by two spine surgeries. Scars from the injury and surgery tethered a large nerve root in my spine, causing severe pain any time I was not lying down. The severe pain lasted four and a half years, and I continue to experience chronic pain, though it is no longer debilitating.

14. Lewis Mumford, *The Myth of the Machine: The Pentagon of Power* (New York: Harcourt Brace Jovanovich, 1970), 435.

15. Søren Kierkegaard, *The Sickness unto Death: A Christian Psychological Exposition for Upbuilding and Awakening*, ed. Howard V. Hong and Edna H. Hong, vol. 19, *Kierkegaard's Writings* (Princeton, New Jersey: Princeton University Press, 1983), 45.

16. Th. Göran Tunevall, "Postoperative Wound Infections and Surgical Face Masks: A Controlled Study," *World Journal of Surgery* 15 (1991): 383–87, https://doi.org/10.1007/BF01658736.

17. My colleague and friend Paul Alexander has compiled a helpful summary of the research studies on masks for the Brownstone Institute: "More than 150 Comparative Studies and Articles on Mask Ineffectiveness and Harms," Brownstone Institute, December 20, 2021, https://brownstone.org/articles/more-than-150-comparative-studies-and-articles-on-mask-ineffectiveness-and-harms/.

18. Zachary J. Madewell et al., "Household Transmission of SARS-CoV-2: A Systematic Review and Meta-Analysis," *JAMA Network Open*, December 14, 2020, https://jamanetwork.com/journals/jamanetworkopen/fullarticle/2774102.; Shiyi Cao et al., "Post-Lockdown SARS-CoV-2 Nucleic Acid Screening in Nearly Ten Million Residents of Wuhan, China," *Nature Communications* 11, no. 5917 (2020), https://doi.org/10.1038/s41467-020-19802-w.

19. Giorgio Agamben, *Where Are We Now: The Pandemic as Politics* (London: Rowman & Littlefield, 2021), 94.

20. Merriam-Webster.com Dictionary, s.v. "faceless," https://www.merriam-webster.com/dictionary/faceless.

21. C. S. Lewis, *Till We Have Faces: A Myth Retold* (New York: HarperOne, 2017).

22. Denise Sosa (@DeniseSo718), "Hong Kong: people are cutting down facial recognition towers," Twitter, May 3, 2022, 10:30 p.m., https://twitter.com/DeniseSo718/status/1521678543796817920.

23. Russell A. Berman, "State of Emergency," *First Things*, no. 324 (June/July 2022), https://www.firstthings.com/article/2022/06/state-of-emergency.

24. Aaron Kheriaty (@akheriaty), "Hey @elonmusk, can you also buy the WHO? It is currently owned by Bill Gates," Twitter, April 19, 2022, 12:59 p.m., https://twitter.com/akheriaty/status/1516461418022727680.

25. Elon Musk (@elonmusk), "I love Pinball Wizard!" Twitter, April 19, 2022, 10:52 p.m., https://twitter.com/elonmusk/status/1516610727641063425.

26. *Schmitt & Landry v. Biden*, no. 22-1213 (W.D. La. 2022), https://ago.mo.gov/docs/default-source/press-releases/mo-la-v-biden-filed-petition.pdf?sfvrsn=3d20bca5_2.

27. "Missouri Attorney General Files Motion for Preliminary Injunction in Lawsuit Challenging Social-Media Censorship," Eric Schmitt: Missouri Attorney General, June

14, 2022, https://ago.mo.gov/home/news/2022/06/14/missouri-attorney-general-files-motion-for-preliminary-injunction-in-lawsuit-challenging-social-media-censorship.

28. Anna Kaplan, "Biden Weighs Public Health Emergency for Abortion Access—Here's What That Means," *Forbes*, July 10, 2022, https://www.forbes.com/sites/annakaplan/2022/07/10/biden-weighs-public-health-emergency-for-abortion-access-heres-what-that-means/.

29. Christian Bjørnskov and Stefan Voigt, "You Don't Always Get What You'd Expect—on Some Unexpected Effects of Constitutional Emergency Provisions," SSRN, June 3, 2018, https://ssrn.com/abstract=3189749.

30. Robert W. Malone, "The Illusion of Evidence-Based Medicine," Who is Robert Malone (Substack), March 28, 2022, https://rwmalonemd.substack.com/p/the-illusion-of-evidence-based-medicine?s=r.

31. John P. A. Ioannidis, "Why Most Published Research Findings Are False," *Public Library of Science Medicine*, August 30, 2005, https://doi.org/10.1371/journal.pmed.0020124.

32. Václav Havel, "Politics and Conscience," in *The Czech Reader*, ed. Jan Bažant et al. (Durham: Duke University Press, 2010).

33. Ibid.

34. Simone Weil, *The Need for Roots*, trans. Arthur Wills (London: Routledge, 2002), 11.

35. Ibid., 27.

36. Augusto Del Noce, *The Age of Secularization*, trans. Carlo Lancelloti (Montreal: McGill-Queen's University Press, 2017), 31.

37. Weil, *The Need for Roots*, 43.

38. Ibid., 97.

39. Ibid., 119.

40. Ibid., 47.

41. Giambattista Vico, *The New Science of Giambattista Vico*, trans. Thomas Goddard Bergin and Max Harold Fisch (Ithaca, New York: Cornell University Press, 1948), 382.

42. Weil, *The Need for Roots*, 241.

43. "Aaron Kheriaty, MD—Full Interview—Planet Lockdown," Source Peertube, February 2022, https://tube.source.news/w/3dc44ef7-d699-4bca-b2f9-6e12d8c6be1b.

Epilogue: Seattle, 2030

1. Note to the reader: except for the fictional medications (Reverie, Keen, Fulsome, and Neurontgen), all the technology described in this epilogue is already available, even if it has not yet been adopted for widespread use. I speculate here on where this technology, deployed by the biomedical security state, will lead society, but the technology itself is not science fiction.

2. Zeger van der Wal and Yifei Yan, "Could Robots Do Better Than Our Current Leaders?" World Economic Forum, October 17, 2018, https://www.weforum.org/agenda/2018/10/could-robot-government-lead-better-current-politicians-ai/.

3. Cf. Dmitry Kireev et al., "Continuous Cuffless Monitoring of Arterial Blood Pressure via Graphene Bioimpedance Tattoos," *Nature Nanotechnology*, June 20, 2022, https://doi.org/10.1038/s41565-022-01145-w.

4. Albert Bourla, CEO of Pfizer, explained the technology of electronic compliance pills in his talk to the World Economic Forum in 2018. The video is available at kalibhakta, "Albert Bourla at World Economic Forum 2018 Is Excited about Electronic Compliance Pills," YouTube, December 28, 2021, https://www.youtube.com/watch?v=1NR1b2NmD4A.

5. Cf. "Peter Schwartz," SalesForce, https://www.salesforce.com/au/blog/authors/peter-schwartz.

6. Microsoft Research, "Programming DNA," YouTube, September 20, 2016, https://youtu.be/sL2I8Fqu9HI.

7. Cf. "Agile Nations Charter," Government of Canada, https://www.canada.ca/en/government/system/laws/developing-improving-federal-regulations/modernizing-regulations/agile-nations.html.

Index

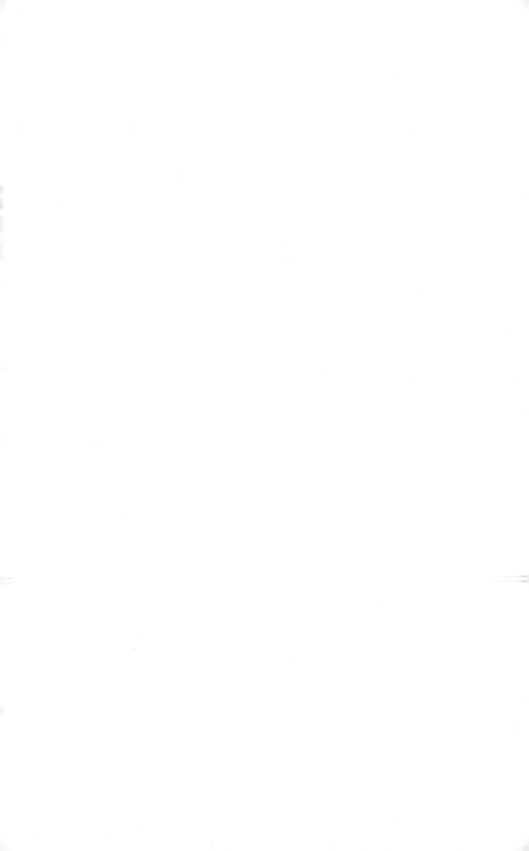